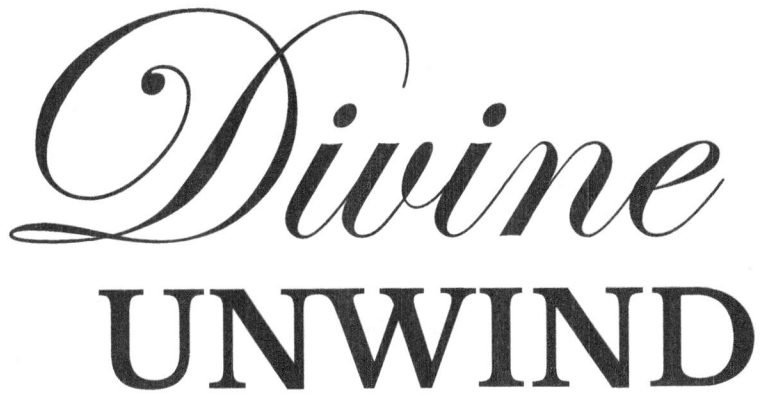

Divine UNWIND

LINDA ANNA

Copyright © 2019 Linda Anna

Divine UNWIND

All rights reserved. No part of this publication may be reproduced, distributed, or transmitted in any form or by any means, including photocopying, recording, or other electronic or mechanical methods, without the prior written permission of the publisher, except in the case of brief quotations embodied in critical reviews and certain other noncommercial uses permitted by copyright law. For permission requests, write to the publisher, addressed "Attention: Permissions Coordinator," at info@beyondpublishing.net

Quantity sales special discounts are available on quantity purchases by corporations, associations, and others. For details, contact the publisher at the address above.

Orders by U.S. trade bookstores and wholesalers. Email info@ BeyondPublishing.net

The Beyond Publishing Speakers Bureau can bring authors to your live event. For more information or to book an event contact the Beyond Publishing Speakers Bureau speak@BeyondPublishing.net

The Author can be reached directly BeyondPublishing.net/ AuthorLindaAnna

Manufactured and printed in the United States of America distributed globally by BeyondPublishing.net

New York | Los Angeles | London | Sydney

ISBN Hardcover: 978-1-949873-01-6

ISBN Softcover: 978-1-947256-33-0

Table of Contents

Foreword	07
Section 1 - Breathing	25
Day 1 No Time Like The Present	27
Day2 Our Busy Lives	29
Day 3 Fighting Fatigue	32
Day4 Why Worry?	34
Section 2 - Freeing the Back	39
Day 5 Body Break	42
Day 6 Get Yourself a Piece of Peace	44
Day 7 All Twisted Up	47
Day 8 An Attitude of Gratitude	50
Day 9 My Friend Fear	52
Section 3 - Releasing the Muscles of the Front	55
Day 10 Emerge	58
Day 11 Keep Moving	61
Section 4 - Releasing muscles of the Waist and Trunk Rotation	65
Day 12 Getting Unstuck	68
Day 13 What You Owe Your Child, Yourself	73
Day 14 Expectation	78
Day 15 More Out of You	80
Day 16 Meditation on a Mediocre Life	83
Day 17 Shallow and Deep	87

Section 5 - Shoulders — 91
    Day 18 A Perfectly Imperfect You — 94

Section 6 - Hips and Legs — 99
    Day 19 What I Would Teach My Younger Self — 101
    Day 20 Thoughts on Not Losing Your Cool — 106
    Day 21 The Art of Solitude — 109
    Day 22 No Bad Days — 113
    Day 23 Mastering the Divine Unwind — 117
    Day 24 Two Secrets to the Divine Unwind — 121

Section 7 - Neck and Shoulders — 125
    Day 25 Thinking Younger Throughout the Day — 127
    Day 26 The Dirty Little Temptation — 130
    Day 27 Resting by Working Harder — 134
    Day 28 Pandiculation — 137
    Day 29 Miracles Are the Everyday Stuff of God — 143
    Day 30 Grounding — 146

Foreword

My first experience with Linda Anna came in a conversation about sacred things. I had known beforehand that Linda was a deep thinker and would shake up the way I thought. I also understood her body of work to involve the relationship between the physical body and one's spirit or soul. I was aching to have a discussion like that.

What I wasn't prepared for was the effect she was to have on my lifelong sacred journey.

As humans, we all share a common desire to make sense of things. Why are we here? What are we to do today? What is our relationship with one another? I have spent a lifetime wrestling with these questions.

We also share one other reality. Every day, we are getting a moment older. We were all born to die, and not one among us will fail in reaching that end. Our bodies grow slower, our minds dim, and one day, unless we are hit by a truck first, we will lay down on the grass, out of breath and fade away.

As we age, our physical bodies lose their bloom. We are surprised to see a face in the mirror lacking the youth we feel in our souls no longer dancing in our eyes.

Linda Anna is eternally young. She has discovered the secret that the creator Source is not a cranky old soul, but rather the fountain of sacred youth, the elixir of enthusiasm with the power to transform life's most ordinary moments. Linda reconnects us with our youthful passions and reminds us how to think and move about in the ways that were so natural to us when we were young.

As the reader, you must want desperately what Linda has to tell you. You need harken back to a day when you could not wait to get out of bed in the morning. When walking was too slow, and you ran everywhere. A time when you laughed a lot, because life was always surprising you. When you never asked why you were alive or what you should do, because you were already doing it.

Linda Anna is about to reconnect you to the enthusiasm of your youth, which has been buried in your soul for a very long while.

You have to want this bad. You will have to forget much of what you think you know. Your desire to feel the exuberance of your youth needs to be greater than your desire to hold on to old ideas. Your ache to feel a bounce in your step again needs to swell into a thirst only becoming young once more can satisfy.

Divine Unwind is about to become your answer to the question, "What is the most important book you have ever read?"

You will have Linda Anna to thank.

It's time for you to come out and play.

Thom Black
Former Executive Pastor
Chicago Megachurch Willow Creek Community Church
Creator, The Amazing Adventures of Harry Moon

Divine UNWIND

A child kicks its legs rhythmically
through excess, not absence, of life.
Because children have abounding vitality,
because they are in spirit fierce and free,
therefore, they want things repeated and unchanged.
They always say, "Do it again,"
and the grown-up person does it again
until he is nearly dead.

For grown-up people are not strong enough
to exult in monotony. But perhaps God is strong enough.
It is possible that God says every morning,
"Do it again," to the sun;
and every evening, "Do it again," to the moon.

It may not be automatic necessity that makes all daisies alike:
it may be that God makes every daisy separately,
and has never got tired of making them.
It may be that He has the eternal appetite of infancy;
for we have sinned and grown old,
and our Father is younger than we.

G.K. Chesterton

WHEN I AM ALONE, I DANCE

I resisted writing this book for a very long time. I was so engaged in my own life journey that it was hard to pop my head out of the ground long enough to wave a snapshot of what I had found.

Somewhere along my path, life's important questions became personal to me. I wanted more than to simply help another find their way. I wanted to help myself. How could I truthfully be present in the life of another if I wasn't authentically present in my own?

I have always known the presence of God in my life. Ever since I was a child, I knew there was something out there, and that He loved me, whatever that meant. However, I walked away from God at 14 years old when my family uprooted from San Diego to Florida. We happily lived on a boat: my mother father, brother, and sheep dog. It was fun, but shallow. One of my happiest memories was on that boat, not a care in the world in my swimsuit lying down with the warm eighty degree wind blowing across my suntanned skin. This felt like heaven.

I plodded along my path away from God and followed the men in my life, wandering further and further away from the God of my youth. I loved adventure, and put much of my energy into having fun, dancing, tennis, skiing, rollerblading, windsurfing—anything with a physical challenge and speed. I felt myself increasingly addicted to love and helplessly searching for love in all the wrong places. I felt isolated in the relationships and losing my identity, as I was always enmeshed with the current man in my life, and worst of all, getting older and running out of time to live the life I had always dreamed of.

I wish there was a day or an idea or a moment when it all changed, but it wasn't that way for me. It was more like someone was slowly turning a dimmer switch, and my thinking was becoming illuminated by degrees. It was an awakening I could not have determined on my own, because every step of my journey was unexpected.

I do know, looking back, what was happening inside of me that created the opportunity for my new sight. There were a series of horrific events when I finally decided to search for the love I had lost. My first love of my youth. The love I had previously was not love at all, but a needy codependent feeling type of love. I longed for something deeper; I believe God has created this longing in each one of us. I cultivated a hunger for a new sound and began listening to my inner voice of wisdom. I began protecting myself from the voices of others always telling me what to do with my life and began listening to the still small voice within. As my heart began to swell with this newfound love—a holy love—it began to overflow in me, and I was able to let go of judging every idea or person that wasn't like me and began to love them all with this new kind of love. Agape.

Most importantly, I made myself available for the Designer, the Source of all there is, to reintroduce himself to me. Over time, every part of who I am became reignited by His enthusiasm for me. I came to understand myself in a way that I had never known before. I discovered I had been overwhelmingly loved by my Designer all these years without my knowing.

All this was happening as I began to get older. Every sunrise added another day. My body was realizing the effects of age while my thinking and interior life seemed to be getting younger. It was a tension no one had warned me about. I could feel a returning, child-like energy flowing from someplace deep inside, against the new aches and pains of an aging body.

But something else was going on. I was experiencing a new connection to the love of my life, the Source of my being, and the well-spring of my youthful enthusiasm. Like Thom said in his foreword, I had rediscovered a bounce in my step that I had lost, and I seemed to be pushing back on the natural aging many of my friends were experiencing.

It was important that this vitality I was coming to know make its way into my work with clients and students, first though my personal training at the gym and teaching classes to benefit the health of others, and later through my Hanna Somatic Training, which was the turning point in my life of discovering the youth from within. I sought out the best thinking and practices of others who had, likewise, discovered the magic of resurrecting the energy of our youth. I was amazed how many had gone before me, how much had been written and testified to regarding what I was just now uncovering. I became a steadfast student of Hanna Somatic Education with a desire to learn how to transfer our eternal youthfulness into not only how we think, but into how we move. I began an intentional divine unwind of my life and everything I thought I had believed and reinvested myself into helping those around me become young again.

COME EMPTY

As I have become a little younger every day, I understand there is something that connects every soul who dares open this door. As you turn the page, you are committing to leaving your past behind.

There is a lot back there behind you, and moving forward is not something that is done lightly. For many, the value of this book is contained in the next few words.

You have collected many sounds over your lifetime. Some of you have been abused, whether verbally or physically. You have been disregarded. Lost a love. Known pain. Experienced financial hardship. Grief. Loss of opportunity. Confusion. Hopelessness. Failures of every possible sort. Words like "you can't," "you won't," and "you never will" ring in your ears. Others have spent a lifetime constructing a life that has all the right questions to all the wrong answers, with a rigidity that never, ever entertains a new thought.

Whomever you are, we stand inside this doorway together in agreement. As we pass through, we are leaving behind, as much as we are able, the sounds and clutter of our past journey. We are intentionally reinventing ourselves and becoming available to grow again, to see new colors and hear new sounds. The Spirit wants to reconnect you to the enthusiasm of your youth and simply requires that you are available to return to that which you were intended to be. Come with me, but come empty.

Oh yes, one more thing. We are going to do something for those aches and pains you have been experiencing. We are going to address those endless trips to the massage therapist and chiropractor and acupuncturist. I am going to remind you how you fluttered as a child and the exuberance of when you were young. I am going to teach you how to move again.

And when you are alone, when no one is looking, you will dance.

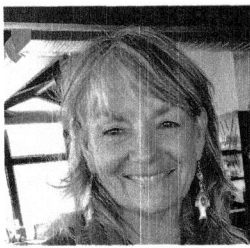

TOMBOY

When I was young, I was a tomboy playing, climbing, swimming, and running around with no fear whatsoever. I fell a lot and would get back up and do it again. My early injuries included a broken wrist in kindergarten, a broken elbow in sixth grade, numerous sprained ankles, bursitis in my left shoulder in high school from swimming, and a knee injury from snow skiing at eighteen.

My life-changing accident was a head injury at age twenty-four slipping on water coming out of a pool. My head bounced off the tile floor, and I went into convulsions. My head was torqued thirty percent to the right. I have been told many times that I should have died from what has happened to my body.

My back has troubled me all of my adult life. I had tried numerous chiropractors over the years, EFT, ART, had orthodics, tried massage, stretching, and every kind of exercise routine, to no avail. When I began to work with the motions and thinking behind somatic movements, my relationship with my body changed.

I felt changes almost immediately with renewed strength in my neck and upper shoulders. Within four weeks, I could see my posture being transformed. My body became more limber each month as the aging of my muscles reversed.

I owe my new-found vitality to my somatic movements. Upon awakening in the morning, I immediately begin my movements, which allow for fluid movement all day long. If I need to work on the computer for more than an hour, I will take a break and do some movements on the floor that allow me to work longer with less strain and fatigue. I finish my day in the evening with my somatic movements, and they relax me from the day's stresses.

At sixty years young, I am weight training, hiking, biking, dancing, playing guitar, and singing. I've also added songwriting and painting to the mix.

I am young again.

Let's open the doorway together.

Your younger self is waiting.

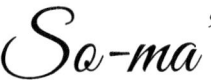

Origin late 19th century: from Greek soma "body"

The living body—the one you sense and feel with all its aliveness.

SOMATIC MOVEMENTS

The somatic movements described in Divine Unwind are movements our bodies did when we were younger. They are not stretches.

We have been designed to move in a manner that is best understood when we examine the movements of children.

A child under the age of twelve moves in many different ways. But is there more to their movement than simply playing? Yes, their movements come naturally, but they are intelligent. These intrinsic movements keep their bodies flexible, coordinated, strong, and resilient. They are in motion made fluid by performing flexible rotations unknowingly all day long. This is by design.

As a child ages, their movements slow down. They become stiffer and stiffer with age. They leave much of their childish movements behind.

Throughout history, many have sought to reconnect aging humans with the movements of their youth. For example, Dr. Thomas Hanna was a genius in this field. He definitely got a download back in the seventies, and I chose to learn this specific work, because by far, he had captured the essence and, particularly, the recipe that divinely unwinds the whole body from head to toe.

He developed "Hanna Somatic Education", which is a series of movement patterns that are based on youthful, intrinsic movements I believe designed into us to keep us limber and flexible. These movements aid in relieving pain, stiffness, fatigue, aging in the muscles, posture, and enhance performance in sports and physical activities.

Devoting oneself to learning and applying these movement patterns will help you stay limber and flexible as your body ages. Your muscles will change, becoming strengthened and longer, relaxed and more comfortable.

Once realized, somatics will enable you to slow down, relax, and breathe deep.

Committing yourself to these youthful movements –along with the inspiration from the devotionals—will renew your body, mind, and spirit.

I will take you there. Come along with me.

Definitions:

The Sensory-Motor Cortex

This part of the brain is between your ears and the top of your head and sends motor information to the muscles and receives sensory information from the muscles. It has unlimited potential for learning new motor plans which create a better sense of balance, coordination, aids in lengthening chronically tight muscles, activating atrophied or inactive muscles and helps you to be successful in your everyday activities.

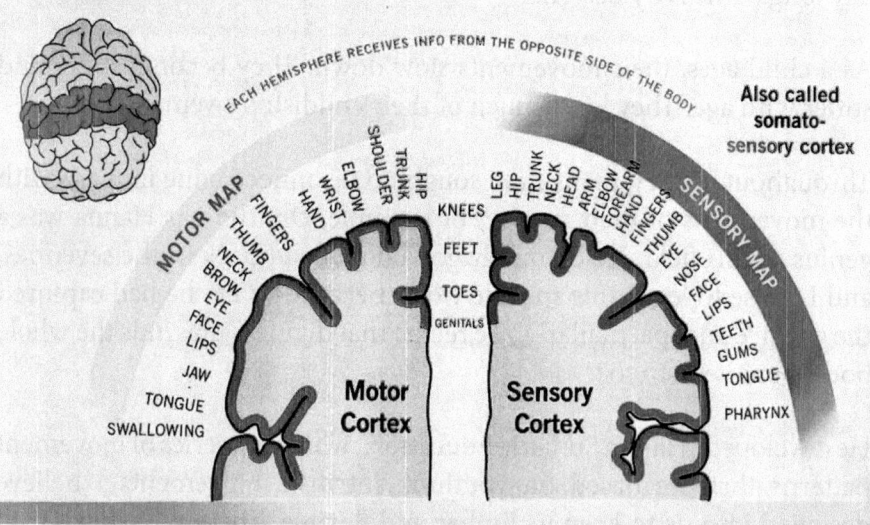

Easy Answers to a FEW SMART QUESTIONS

What is somatic?

The root word '**soma**' means living body, your own first-person perspective of what you sense and feel. Somatic is movement pertaining to the soma, what is right and good for you.

How often should I do somatic movements?

Movements should be performed twice a day for realignment and reprogramming. Habits take twenty-one days to establish. Our bad habits are so ingrained, we need to remind our somas optimally two times per day. Optimally, in the morning to prepare for the activities of the day, and in the evening, to release habitual movements accumulated throughout the day and for better sleep.

How are somatic movements different from chiropractic, acupuncture, or massage?

In most other modalities, the practitioner is working on you, and you are passive. In somatic movements, you are active, and the practitioner is working *with* you to teach you how to re-awaken your sensory-motor system. You are coached on posture, sitting, standing, and walking patterns. You are taught movement patterns to manage on your own towards self-care.

Are somatic movements compatible with physical therapy?

If you are under a doctor's care, always follow their instructions. Physical therapy includes strengthening and stretching exercises. Somatic movements are best done separately, after physical therapy has ended. A physical therapist may only work on the shoulder if specified to do so. A somatic educator is taught to work with the entire body in a holistic way and help correct the core of the problem working from the core to the periphery and helping the student gain awareness in the soma, which may lead to self-correction of habitual movement patterns.

BENEFITS FROM SOMATIC MOVEMENTS

- Relieve pain and stiffness by moving like a child
- Roll back the age of your muscles
- Re-activate your brain and gain motor plans
- Improve muscle memory.
- Become more flexible every year you age
- Improve coordination and skill
- Improve your gait and walking pattern
- Restore function and enhance performance
- Relieve anxiety, fear, and stress
- Improve sense of balance
- Elevate your posture and look taller
- Enjoy a better quality of life and fewer health issues
- Prevent injuries
- Smile more often
- Dance, sing, and play upon request

OUR LANGUAGE

As one grows younger, we return to behavior that was important to us when we were so very young. We want to be thoughtful as we rewind and remember again what once came naturally to us.

Be Mindful: Pay attention to the sensations you are feeling. In somatic movement, you stimulate the part of the brain that receives sensory information and sends out motor information to the muscles. Paying attention to what you are thinking and feeling will awaken you to a new sense of awareness.

Be Focused: Perform your somatic movements isolated from all distractions, including music, phone, and screens. Clutter and noise lessen the effect of your intentional movements.

Be Slow and Deliberate: Moving slowly allows time for feedback to move from muscles to the brain in a motor feedback loop. Fast movements do not contribute to the effect of a somatic movement.

Be Gentle: All movements should be done effortlessly. Straining will keep the muscles from releasing. Do your movements lazily, as if you just woke up.

Be Relaxed: Do not force any movement. No amount of force can relieve the involuntary contractions in your body. If you want to untie a knot, you must look at the cord carefully before gently undoing the tangle. Yanking on the cord will only make the knot tighter.

Be Careful: Somatic movements are not painful. If you perform them slowly and gently, they are completely harmless. Hurting yourself while exercising is unnecessary, harmful, and no fun at all. People who are suffering from sensory-motor amnesia (a lack of awareness of how certain muscles feel) and have severely contracted muscles may feel some soreness when these muscles first begin to lengthen and "remember". By doing the movements consistently, soreness tends to dissipate, and lactic acid (which causes the soreness) may be removed from the muscles. If you feel some pain when doing the movements, back off or decrease the amount of movement and do micro movements. Increase your range of motion later, when you feel more comfortable and confident.

Be Persistent: By doing the movements daily, you are reminding your muscles how to lengthen and relax, eventually gaining an everyday freedom.

Be Patient: Somatic exercises change your entire being by teaching your body and brain. Your retention grows steadily and solidly as you learn new motor plans. Some movements may seem awkward at first, be patient; not looking for a quick fix, but a lasting change in your comfort, range of motion, posture, and general overall function.

THE DIVINE UNWIND AND YOU

You now begin to take seriously the work of staying young. Somatic movements are movements for a lifetime.

The more you do, the more energy you have for the things you love. Children flutter about all day long. That's why they have so much energy.

There is no quick fix. Your retention grows steadily and solidly as you re-learn patterns you had when you were young. Each day adds up to regaining mobility, flexibility, agility, and coordination.

Patience will become your virtue. Your brain has unlimited potential for learning. Your muscles can learn, and it takes time to reverse chronic contractions.

You will feel some changes right away. Some pains may disappear within days. Others, after some time. The effects are cumulative. You get more and more flexible every month you practice your movements.

REMEMBER, NO HARM

All somatic movements are gentle, normal, and organic movements of the muscular skeletal system. If done slowly and easily, they are completely harmless.

If you have severely contracted muscles, do very small movements. Always consult your physician if you have severe pain.

DISCLOSURE

Somatic movement is not a medical treatment, nor is it intended to be a substitute for conventional medical diagnosis or treatment.

Somatics reawakens the neuromuscular system to release chronically contracted painful muscles, and to bring about a better balance in the body. An understanding of somatic movements is for the purpose of learning how to recognize, release, and reverse sensory motor awareness.

CHATTER ABOUT THE DIVINE UNWIND

You have enlightened me as to how to unwind the chronic contractions in my body. With just one session, you identified the problem areas and gave me the right movements to release the tension. I went from months of pain and discomfort and not being able to sit or stand for long periods of time due to hip pain and shooting pain down the legs to complete relief. I had been unable to sleep, due to the pain on both sides. Now, after just one private session and one group session at Moonlight Overlook Park in Encinitas, I am pain-free and fully functional. Mahalo nui loa. Anne

IF YOU CAN BELIEVE IT, YOU CAN DO IT

Do you think you can become young again? Do you believe you have the capacity to grow young and find that magical bounce you remember when you were a child? Do you believe in the restorative powers of play?

Thirty Days To
THE NEW, YOUNGER YOU

The discipline of practicing somatic movements daily can help you turn these intentional actions into habits.

The Thinking Behind Change

A habit is a learned automatic response you do without thinking. Forming your new habit of movement involves multiple steps, including: making a decision to change, initiating the new behavior, and repeating it often.

Turning movements into habits will take a little time. A thirty-day launch can help to get the ball rolling, but it may not be enough to make the lasting change we are looking for. In fact, research suggests it takes an average of sixty-six days for your new movements to become a natural part of your everyday life. Missing one day does not hinder your progress, but the more you miss, the longer it will take for the habits to form.

Take a Whack at Thirty Days

1. It provides the boost you may need to get started in your movements.
2. The daily repetition boosts momentum to return to your movements every day.
3. As you keep going, achieving small successes can help motivate you to keep going.

I want you to understand the stages of change and how thoughtful you need to be as you begin the divine unwind.

Stages of Change

Change is made in small steps or stages. The "pre-contemplation stage" occurs as you begin to think actively about committing yourself to youthful movements. The next stage involves thinking and planning with actual, observable change evolving as new movements are put in place.

It's only in the next stage of repetition that the actual new movements become natural. Interestingly, if the movements are dropped for a while, don't be discouraged. This isn't considered a failure, but rather a predictable part of the whole process of the unwind, and even a specific stage of change, if you don't give up trying. It's considered a part of the process of creating movements that last a lifetime.

Tips for Turning a Movement into a Habit

1. **Tying new movements to a current routine can be useful.** If you read every morning, or sit down with a cup of coffee, fold your intentional movements inside of the routine. Studies have shown that when you are looking to learn or acquire a new behavior, you have a better chance to develop a pattern if you connect it to an existing routine.

Creating sub-routines in the middle of an existing routine can have a greater likelihood of habit formation.

2. **Develop a positive mental attitude toward your movements.** Be excited about them. These movements are not a diet or to remind you that you are getting older. If you don't love the opportunity to spend a few moments with yourself to unlock your youth, it's unlikely you will stick with it very long.

3. **Learning your somatic movements along with supportive friends—in real life or virtually—adds an additional level of support.** Some people find shared activities offer an aspect of mutual encouragement that helps propel them forward.

Begin Your Thirty Days VERY SOON

Many readers find it a challenge to actually begin something. It's always nice to have and work toward a goal. Too often, we look to the future to make such a significant commitment. Divine unwind? Every day? Sounds like a great idea. Think I'll start that after Thanksgiving. Nope. Make that Christmas.

The fundamental flaw in looking toward the future is that the future is just that. The future.

Meanwhile, the advantages of tapping into your youth go unrealized. Another day passes. A tad bit more tired. Shoulder still stiff, elbow achy. We can only hope how it will turn out. We have only one guarantee of what will happen tomorrow. We will be another day older.

But we *do* have control over the present. Your commitment toward a youthful life of movement could begin today.

So, what does your first step toward thirty days of youth look like? First, breathe. Calm yourself down. Quiet your mind and focus on the current moment. Focus on the present and ask yourself if you are ready to do this. Call a friend and invite them to take this thirty-day journey with you.

I believe in you. The thirty-day payoff will change your life.

Your youthful movements are part of your sacred journey, your way back to the garden. They are your path beyond stress and pain, to strength and vitality.

Hope, peace, and joy are within reach. Your movements are my gift to you.

SECTION ONE

Breathing

DAY ONE

No Time Like
THE PRESENT

There is no other time, period.
We only have the moment we are living in.
What's past is past. Can't do anything about it.
All gone. You can't relive what happened yesterday
(I know many people who try).
What's going to happen tomorrow hasn't happened yet,
and who knows if it ever will?
And even if you do wake up tomorrow,
it won't be tomorrow anymore. It will be today.
You know it's true, don't you?
And if you are starting out on this sacred journey with me,
then we probably already agree.
If you have something you want to do,
then when you put the book down, do it.
If you love someone who doesn't know, pick up the phone.
If you love someone who knows, tell them again.
If you did something naughty, go make it right.
If you woke with a dream, figure it out.
If you are living the best life ever, then let everyone know.
Get the point? Your sacred moment is the eternity you were waiting for.
Your opportunity to touch your destiny started five minutes ago.
We want to see you glimmering. The time is now!
Unwind to when you were young.

There was only the present. Tomorrow never came, and it never mattered. The only thing we did was what we wanted to do today. Tomorrow was for all the things we didn't like to do today. We never worried about tomorrow. We were too busy with today.
Come on. We were kids.

MOVEMENT

DIAPHRAGMATIC BREATHING EXERCISE:

Close your eyes and notice if you are breathing or holding your breath. Take a moment to sense your breathing. Notice if your chest is rising and falling or if your breaths are short and fast. Notice if your belly is moving or feels restricted, maybe because of clothing. Many have become accustomed to stress and tight jeans.

Place your right hand on your upper abdomen, and your left hand on your upper chest. As you breathe in, concentrate on the air moving down into the upper abdomen and expanding around the ribs. Think of your belly filling up with air, like a balloon, expanding when you inhale, and deflating when you exhale. The right hand should rise with the inhalation and fall with the exhalation. The chest should remain still, and the breath should be gentle and effortless. Try breathing in and out through the nose. Focus on your breathing becoming smooth and even.

What is Diaphragmatic Breathing?

Also known as belly breathing, it is the way we were designed to breath. Children breathe with their belly. The belly goes out when inhaling, and the belly goes in when exhaling. It is a deeper breathing pattern, using more of the lung capacity and helps relieve stress and deliver nutrients to brain cells. It keeps the nervous system in a calm, restorative state, as opposed to an anxious fight-or-flight state.

Awareness and healthy breathing have a significant effect on health and well-being. Isn't it amazing that one of the most important things you will take away from The Divine Unwind will be something as simple as an awareness of how you breathe?

Establish diaphragmatic breathing as your normal, everyday breathing habit. Eventually, the easy, rhythmic motion of the diaphragmatic breathing will replace the strained, unnatural chest breathing to which you may have become accustomed. Be aware of your breathing pattern throughout the day.

DAY TWO

Our Busy LIVES

"Let me check my calendar."
"I need to check my schedule first."

How many times in a given week do those phrases, or something similar, come out of your mouth? Whose schedule are you on, anyway?

We are frazzled. Our work, our families, our relationships are frayed at the edges. It doesn't matter if you're a career-driven workaholic or a stay-at-home mom: the pace of our world can be a bit much.

If it's not business meetings, it's a church gathering. If it's not taking mom to the doctor or the dog to the vet, it's trying to get the gardening done. It's always something!

All roads seem to lead to stress—the sort of stress that can sneak up on us, hitting us before we even know it's coming. When you feel yourself getting overwhelmed with life and all of its craziness, take the advice of millions of inspirational songs, coffee mugs, books, and self-help gurus: just breathe.

Watch a baby sleep. "Sleeping like a baby" is truer than your realize. When asleep, their breathing is relaxed, casual, and effortless.

Think about that the next time you need to take a moment to just breathe. Think of how babies sleep, tiny humans that are still free from the stress of calendars and schedules. All they have to do is breathe.

Unwind to when you were young.

I was never busy. I was too distracted being a kid. I was preoccupied with figuring out what I wanted to do next. I'll be home at dinnertime.

It's a pretty summer day that lasts a lifetime, and I'm going to get lost in it.

MOVEMENT

SWIMMER'S BREATH EXERCISE:

May help with stress, high blood pressure, anxiety, racing thoughts, or trouble sleeping.

After you've established a smooth, even pattern of breathing, change your breathing by exhaling twice as long as you inhale. Inhale through the nose counting to two or three, then exhale through the nose and count to four or six. Repeat this 10 to 20 times. This exercise establishes a relaxed state in the body and stimulates the parasympathetic nervous system. It is better than counting sheep when it comes to sleeping. Clear your mind from negative thoughts, and focus on your body and the sensations you feel, or meditate on sacred words.

You will keep in perfect peace all who trust in you. Isaiah 26:3

Be anxious for nothing. Instead, pray about everything. Proverbs 4:6

Be thankful.

CHEST BREATHING

When you breathe from your chest, instead of from your belly (diaphragm), you signal your body to prepare for an "emergency". The nervous system changes from parasympathetic to sympathetic. It is like flipping on a light switch. The more stress you have, the more the light switch is on. Chest breathing increases your heart rate and blood pressure, creating a physiological emergency-like state, also referred to as "fight or flight".

This pattern can become habituated in the body and cause many other problems later on, such as insomnia, nervousness, fatigue, heart problems, and asthma.

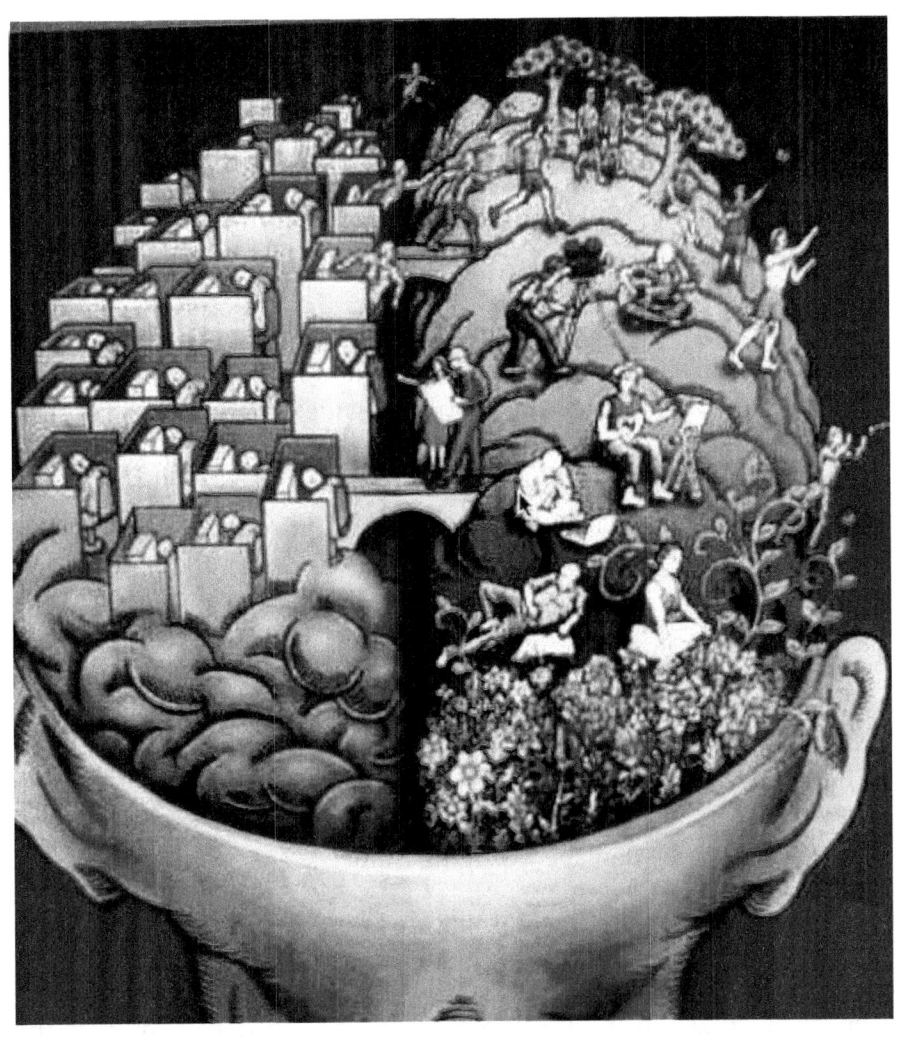

Which part of the brain do you think developed first the right side of the brain or the left side of the brain?

DAY THREE

Fighting FATIGUE

If you've worked in an office setting, you know the importance of having an ergonomically correct workstation. Without a properly put-together workspace, you may start to suffer from a wide variety of health issues: strained eyesight, carpal tunnel syndrome, tendonitis, poor back alignment, and migraines. Studies from the Mayo Clinic suggest sitting behind a computer incorrectly can even lead to serious issues such as high blood pressure and high cholesterol levels.

Even if you are in the peak shape of your life, constant fatigue from being overworked and falling into a slouchy posture behind your desk at work is going to negatively affect your frame. Even if the time at the gym has your exterior looking like a million bucks, your support – your spine, joints, and muscles – are weak. It would be like remodeling a house with the best materials money can buy and then slapping it all together on a water-damaged, sagging frame.

There are some simple steps to fighting fatigue, some of which are so simple that you likely know most of them. Movement is key.

Step Away: Take ten minutes every hour or so to step away from the desk. Take a walk, grab some water or a snack. Step outside to get some fresh air and do one of the breathing exercises—you will feel refreshed.

Improve Your Surroundings: Make sure your workspace is healthy. Check the distance from the screen to your face and that your seat is accommodating and comfortable.

Unwind to when you were young.

I don't remember being tired when I was a child. I absolutely remember being bored. Now that I am an adult, I know what tired is. And I remember being bored. Bored is worse.

MOVEMENT

SOMATIC BREATHING EXERCISE~ *sitting any way*

Perform anywhere when you have neck tension, headache, shoulder tension, or hand tension.

Inhale slowly through the nose, expanding the belly and ribs, allowing the chest to rise (while still breathing in), lift your shoulders to your ears and the elbows away from the body. Exhale in reverse, allowing the shoulders to come down, the elbows into your waist, the arms relax long at your sides, and finally, the belly pulls in. This exercise reduces muscle tension and mental fatigue. It may relieve tension in the neck, upper arms, and thumbs. Practice for 5 minutes or more.

HEALTHY BREATHING

You don't have to be a yogi to breath correctly. We can learn much from our children. Babies and young children breathe with ease. They also move effortlessly and stay stress-free by being in the present. There is a wisdom to their ways. Healthy breathing is achieved by taking deeper breaths from the belly and lower ribs, where the diaphragm is located. You can feel an expansion of the ribs all the way around and into your back.

DAY FOUR

Why WORRY?

"Don't worry, be happy."
-Bobby McFerrin

Remember that song? It was a popular little tune in the 80s, and you could not get the whistling melody out of your head.

The words were irresistible. The message it conveyed was simple and what everyone wanted to hear. "Don't worry, be happy." Incredibly simple, but not nearly as easy as it sounds.

Worrying is a meaningless exercise for human beings. It accomplishes nothing other than upping our anxiety and stress.

There is a rather popular bit of wisdom out of a particular holy writing that goes like this -

"Do not worry about your life, what you will eat or drink; or about your body, what you will wear. Is not life more than food, and the body more than clothes? Look at the birds of the air; they do not sow or reap or store away in barns, and yet your heavenly Father feeds them. Are you not much more valuable than they? Can any one of you by worrying add a single hour to your life?"

Worrying about tomorrow, or even the next hour, is pointless. It assumes that you should have control over all things. You know that is not true.

Doing away with worry is one of the more difficult challenges you face in your divine unwind.

It requires the relinquishing of control and being able to visualize yourself releasing your stress and worries. Think of each of your worries as heavy stones you have been carrying around, weighing you down.

Visualize yourself tossing each of those stones into a river and watching them sink until they disappear completely.

> *"When you live in the past,*
> *with its mistakes and regrets,*
> *it is hard.*
> *I am not there.*
> *My name is not - I WAS.*
> *When you live in the future,*
> *with its problems and fears,*
> *it is hard.*
> *I am not there.*
> *My name is not - I WILL BE.*
> *When you live in this moment,*
> *It is not hard.*
> *I am here.*
> *My name is I AM."*
>
> ***Helen Mallicoat***

Unwind to when you were young.

Did I worry about my life when I was a child? Let me think. I had food every day on the table, a roof over my head, and clothes to wear to school and play in. Nope. I think I was good.

Note; to readers who did not have a nice childhood. The trauma is deep, but God is deeper. Allow Him to dig up the rocks and hard places in your heart and visualize the fertilizer of the spirit refreshing the soil, and friends coming alongside, sprinkling the water.

Look for it, think it, speak it out loud, and your thoughts will become reality.

There is scientific research on this concept.

Check out Dr. Masaru Emoto's Water Experiment, "WORDS ARE POWERFUL".

MOVEMENT

UNWINDING BREATHING EXERCISE~ *standing*

Stand with a wide stance.
Relax the pelvic floor muscles.
Roll the shoulders three times up, back, and down.
Palms inward, bring the arms out and up overhead, lower slowly sighing or sounding *haaaaa*.
Repeat three times.
Palms inward.
Palms forward.
Palms backward.
Cross the arms in front of the body and circle out to the sides three times.
Reach up to one side and down to the other side.
Repeat three times. Go back to work refreshed.
Repeat a positive affirmation or sacred scripture
I am feeling thankful today for _____.

With each breath, say each coworker's name that you are thankful for. Watch things change around work.

"A tranquil heart gives life to the body." Proverbs 14:30

HEALTHY BREATHING:

It keeps the mind and body functioning at its best. Breathing can be calming, relaxing, and help you to de-stress. Healthy breathing lowers blood pressure, heart rate, and helps one focus and sleep better.

MORE CHATTER:

"Somatics has been a real lifesaver for me! I had lost about forty pounds, and was working out vigorously two hours a day. However, I was constantly plagued by aches and pains, particularly in my back and shoulders.

"I went to a chiropractor once a week for several months, and after hundreds of dollars, found I was just wasting my money. I met Linda and started incorporating somatic movements into my daily routine. Everything changed. I was able to do my workouts with much less pain, and to recover from vigorous activities—like snow skiing—without having to see a doctor. I have been able to listen to my body and have become more aware of my posture and balance. I now incorporate at least five minutes of movements first thing in the morning, and do two longer routines during the week to re-educate my muscles."
Joanne Olson

SECTION TWO

Freeing THE BACK

Releasing
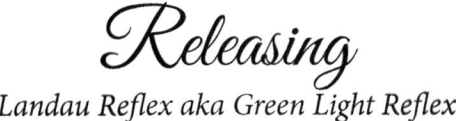
Landau Reflex aka Green Light Reflex

MILITARY-TYPE POSTURE

The posture looks straight, but not relaxed. This person may lock their knees, tightening extensor muscles throughout the entire body, including the neck and back.

Things that may cause this posture to habituate: A-type personality – go, go, go, when sometimes, you should stop. Anxiety, deadlines, alarms. Ballerinas and gymnasts may get this posture from harsh training.

Strengths: Back muscles are strong.

Weakness: Abdominals and stomach muscles – person may not be able to engage their abdominals very well until muscles of the back are released. Flexion of the spine is difficult, making it difficult to reach one's toes.

DAY FIVE

Body BREAK!

The world that is waiting for you this morning is moving kind of fast. It's wound real tight.

Our relationships and how we communicate doesn't help matters. We live on our screens. I know that half of you readers have checked for texts twice since you started reading this book. I know.

It just doesn't stop. There seems to be no getting away from it. And no one seems to be immune.

Many tell me that they are sick of it and are getting sick FROM it. The overstimulation is exhausting and is creating any number of anxious reactions.

I give myself intentional body breaks throughout the day. I need the personal escape. All somatic movements affect the nervous system, movements you and I can easily do just about any time of the day.

Taking these somatic body breaks during the day can lessen tension in the nervous system. It's like taking a vacation in your own hometown.

When you redirect your brain towards things that make you feel grateful, thankful, or blessed, anxiety tends to disappear.

Unwind to when you were young.

I do remember the anxiousness of not knowing when I was a child what would happen with the dentist? New school year? Problems with a friend? I know it helped me to talk to someone who seemed to understand. That seemed to matter.

MOVEMENT

ARCH and FLATTEN

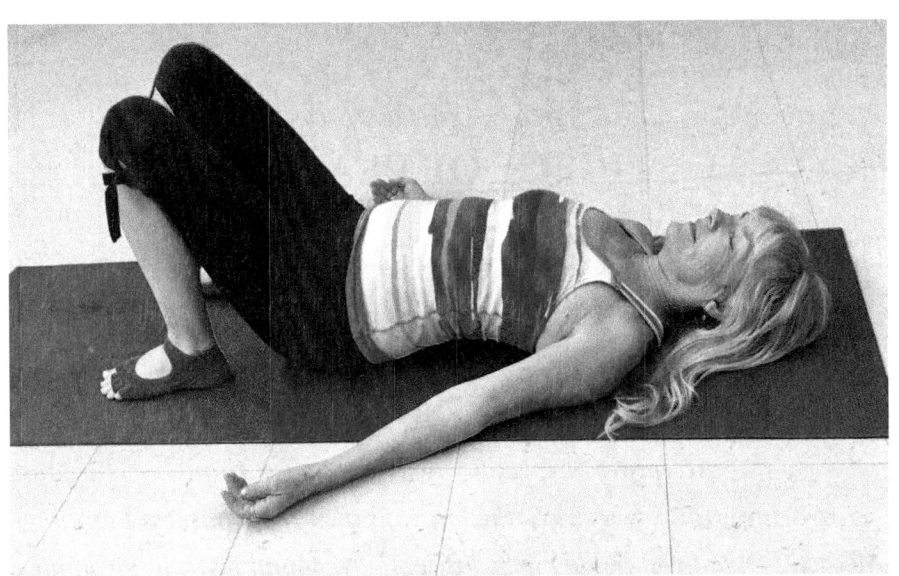

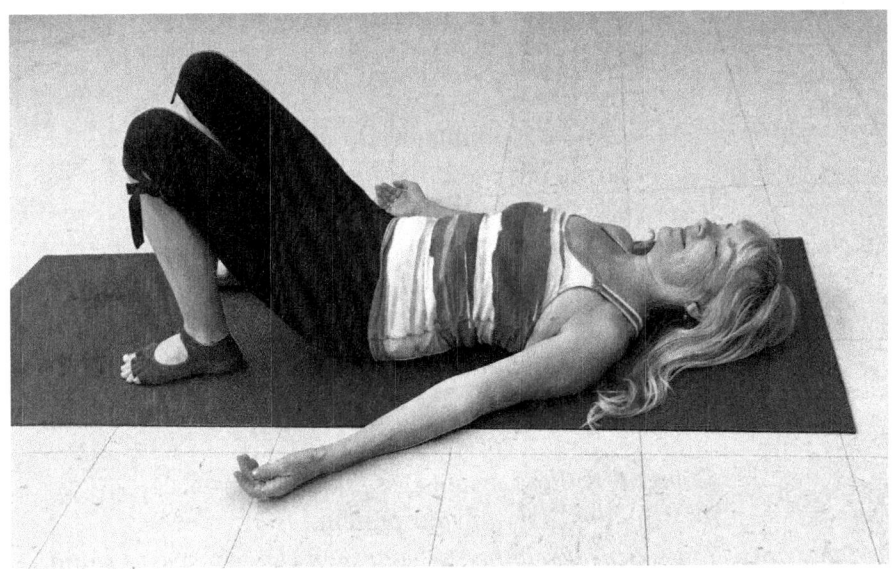

DAY SIX

Get Yourself a
PIECE OF PEACE

I love these lyrics to a Phil Kaeggy song. I know only God can give you peace, but we can find it near.

*Grace~ gracious love
Reaching out to take me as I am,
Accepting~ expecting I will do the best I can.
Caring~ You cover me clothed in your own righteousness I am.
Exactly~ what you made me by grace, I have found favor in the lamb.*

Cover me~Cover me~ Cover me

*Mercy~ made free to me
Eternal life a gift that has no end
Receiving~ believing in the mercy you extend
Cover me~ you cover me, clothed in your own righteousness I stand
Your mercy has made me part of your salvation army band.*

Heart to God~Hand to man~Saved to serve

*Peaceful sleep
Enjoyed by those whose eyes find rest in you.
Adoring the Glory of your presence is in view.
Cover me~You cover me, clothed in your own righteousness I stand.
Eternally~you made me.*

Salvation Army band

Phil Kaeggy

Over these thirty days, we are going to find the divine and the peace that eludes us.

During your divine unwind, I want you to take pride at having achieved something that you never expected. Quietness in the body is an achievement.

A peaceful heart gives life to the body. **Proverbs 14:30**

As you make progress in your youthful movements and find your body unwinding, I want to celebrate anything that represents a move toward your youthful self. Notice things like the energy in your body, the length, width, and temperature. Even minor relief of pain is something, and that is so much more than nothing.

Master peace ~ the Art of God

Unwind to when you were young.

Remember the most beautiful sunset you ever saw. Take a moment and reflect. Notice the sounds~what do you smell? Salty air? What do you feel? Sand between your toes? Take five minutes. My favorite was living on the boat in San Diego. It was glorious. Hot pink, puffy, cotton candy clouds sat on the horizon, and I will never forget that most magnificent sunset; I can go back there any time.

We are here, enjoying the NOW.

Be aware of peacefulness.

MORE CHATTER:

"Ever since I was a kid, I have played many sports. I focused on power lifting and bodybuilding-style exercises. As a result, my body has developed some chronic pain and poor posture. With Divine Unwind, I have the ability to relax tight muscles and realign my posture without having to suffer the pain of another person manipulating my body.

"I use somatic movements to align my body before I lift weights or do high intensity cardiovascular exercise. My body naturally goes into better

alignment when performing exercises. It has reduced the workload on my dominant side and redistributed the load evenly with an incredible decrease in pain." **Chris Wells**

MOVEMENT
ARCH AND CURL

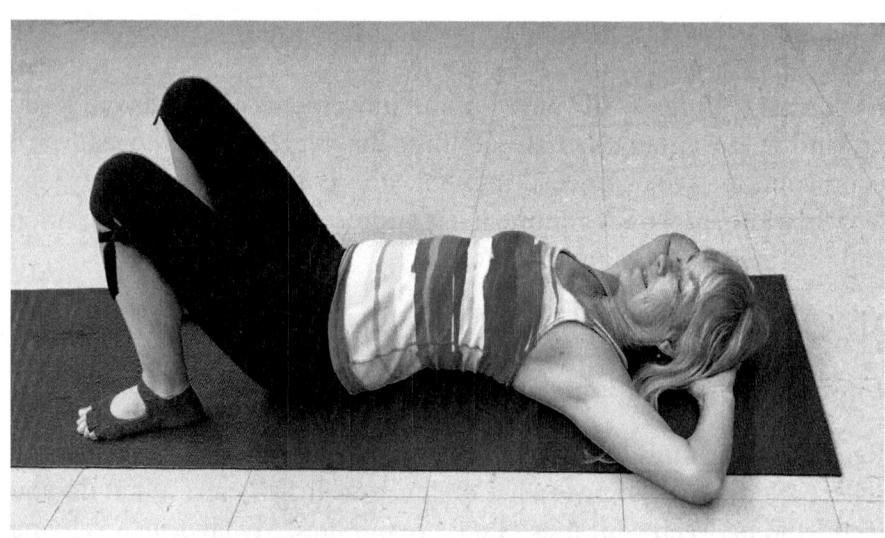

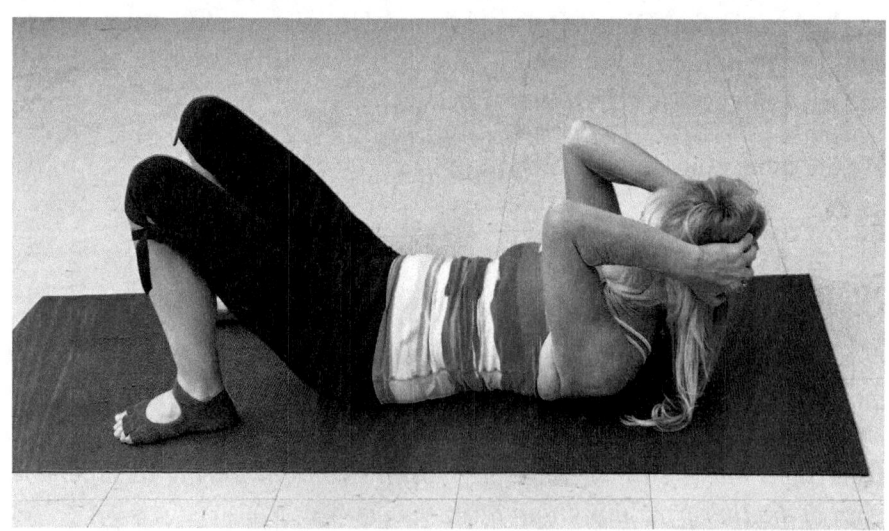

DAY SEVEN

All TWISTED UP

I was traveling with my best friend and teacher from school on a bus to Park City, Utah. In those days, we could ski all day nonstop, barely even pausing for lunch. Well, near the end of the day, wouldn't you know it, I fell in the shape of a pretzel with one ski and foot behind the other, terribly wrenching my knee. I limped to the ski lift for the last run of the day and skied fine. Wouldn't you know it, I couldn't walk for a week. Man, was I crazy.

Physical traumas to the body can be challenging to overcome. From a simple sprained ankle to a wrenched knee or broken back, the body handles traumas in a variety of different ways. Fortunately, with most injuries and setbacks, your brain and nervous system can be "reeducated", making recovery easier for some.

People handle physical traumas differently. For instance, after a physical trauma to the body, some may feel defeated if they have a difficult time recovering. This is especially true of those who are used to living a very active lifestyle. It is hard to accept that your way of life may very well be forever changed.

Some people have strong traumatic reflexes that keep them from making a full recovery. One might be hesitant to put weight on a previously broken leg. An athlete might be hesitant to get back on the field after an injury took them out of the game.

You may have tried everything from physical therapists, to acupuncturists, to chiropractors and more, but nothing seems to give you the exuberance and mobility you once had.

Thoughts like, "I must be getting old," or, "I guess those days are over," may creep in.

Remember that the divine unwind has been created to move you backward to a season of your life when your movements were without restraint. Your somatic movements will release the trauma and muscles that are stuck in habituated patterns. When muscles are stuck, they can be stiff and painful. But we are learning a new way to overcome.

You are becoming your own life coach, listening to the needs of your body and training where it should go.

Unwind to when you were young.

I was in Germany to visit my uncle Erwin, my favorite person in the whole world. We were skiing in Mayrhofen ski resort in Austria. In the morning for breakfast we Enjoyed fresh rolls, butter and cheese and milk from the cows. The snow glistened. I wasn't used to skiing in powder. When I fell I landed with both knees down in the deep snow and my skis and feet above the snow in a knock-kneed position. I kept skiing! Having fun was my number one priority!

MOVEMENTS

PELVIC ROLL

Lie on your back with knees bent.

- A. Lift the right hip up pushing the right foot down, relax the pelvis.

    Repeat 3 times.

- B. Lift the left hip pushing the left foot down, relax to Centr. Repeat 3 times

- C. Alternate, pushing the right foot down and tilting the right hip up to the ceiling, rocking to the other side pushing the left foot down tilting the left hip towards the ceiling. And rocking gently side to side, 6 times

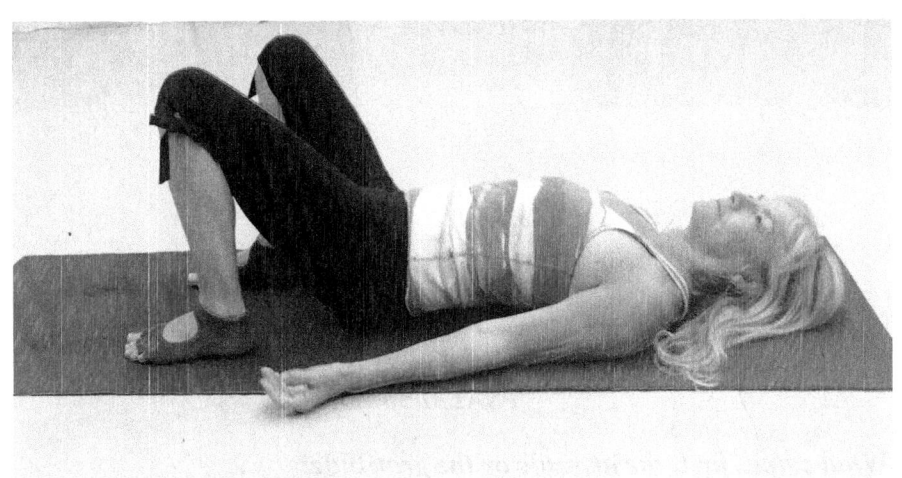

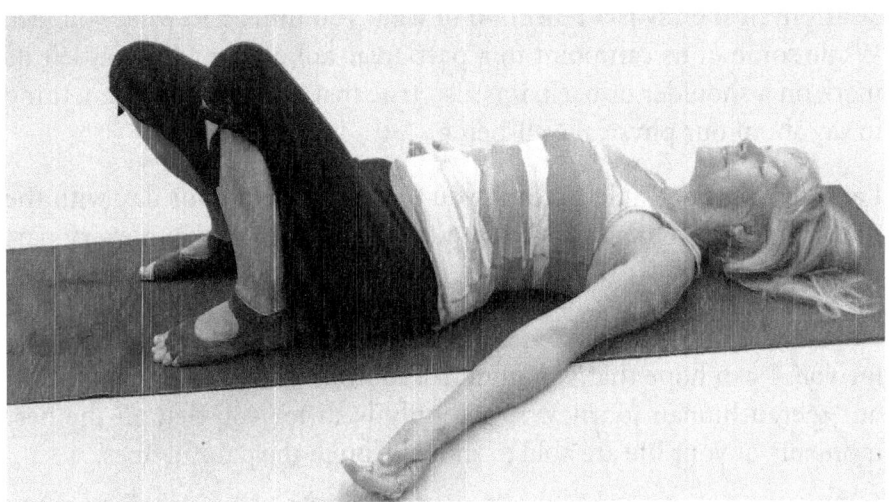

DAY EIGHT

An Attitude of GRATITUDE

"The one who offers thanksgiving as his sacrifice glorifies me."
PSALM 50

What comes first, the attitude or the gratitude?

Your physical body is a reflection of what you think and what you feel. While some of us can point to a particular fall or moment that left its mark on a shoulder or back, it is also true that our heart has something to say about our physical well-being.

I am thrilled to be able to teach you to flutter about your day with the movements of a child. I know the difference it will make in every part of your life.

I also know that when it comes to matters of the heart, I can only hope for you. I can hope that you understand how remarkable it is to be on our sacred human journey. I can only wish for you that all the best moments of your life are able to shine through the painful ones.

I pray that the wisdom of your years creates an ability to love before you judge and to hug before you hate.

Unwinding your life returns you to the enthusiasm and expectation we had so many years ago, that each day, something magical might happen, if we stayed awake long enough.

Unwind to when you were young.

We were traveling in our motorhome and my dad would always take the short cut which turned out to take two hours longer. My brother and I would ride up in the top of the camper watching all the excitement. We drove into the wee hours of the night and when we would arrive at the campground it looked very creepy and spooky. The next day we would wake up in paradise.

MOVEMENT

LIFT UPS

    A. Lift elbow three times.

    B. Lift the head and look over your shoulder three times.

    C. Lift the elbow and opposite leg up simultaneously and lower three to six times slowly, until your entire back and legs relax.

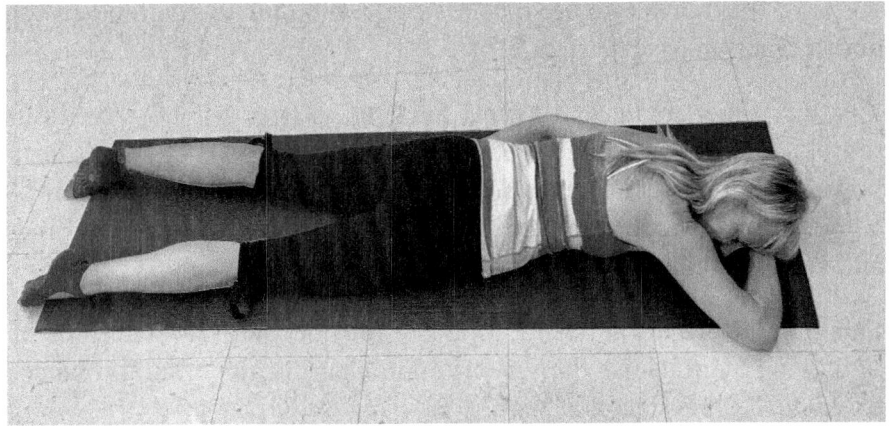

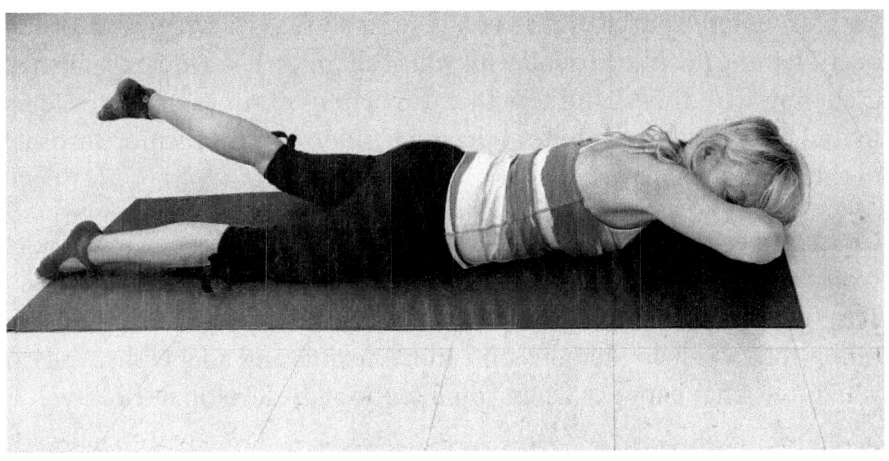

DAY NINE

My Friend FEAR

We're all afraid of something. Not measuring up, pain, getting old.

It could be something as simple as the dark or as personal as a trigger that reminds you of some past fall, accident or terror.

We have this reflex and are helpless against it. Our startle reflex is the body's reaction to fear.

This fear thing matters. It affects us. It takes over our body and our muscles tighten and infects how we feel. Ever hold a balloon and it pops in your hands? The sense of being startled causes your body to automatically flex, in an attempt to protect itself. Do that enough times and you are a mess inside.

This reflex is a natural born into us but may become habitual in many individuals. Adults use the sensory motor part of the brain to manage this and all other flavors of fear.

This fear entered our lives at a young age, as soon as we were aware of our peers. It hung out like a friend with you at all times. It is a lifelong journey grappling with this friend fear that can grip us at times or motivate us to find the sparkle and shine at the other side. This motivation leads us to the adventure.

Getting over these fears can be uncomfortable for some. Most adults typically do things they are good at and don't try new things as they age. They prefer to stay in a comfortable little bubble and avoid the very things that will help them become more flexible and adaptable. And do you know what happens when you intentionally develop flexibility?

You release your fears from the inside out.

Their is no fear in love, for perfect love casts out all fear. 1 John 4:18

Doing something new feels awkward at first. It makes us feel vulnerable and uneducated. But studies have shown that learning stimulates brain growth and new muscle length, reversing aging in the muscles.

Some have a fear of moving a previously injured area. It is our way of guarding the injury site. All muscles, tendons, ligaments and joints have sensory nerve receptors, the sites that send information to the central nervous system and then to the sensory-motor cortex. In other words, your body remembers each trauma.

This sort of fear creates tightness on one side of the body while also causing body's the trauma reflex. This often causes tightness in areas such as, but not limited to: the jaw, neck, shoulders, back, waist, hips and feet. Release this reflex in chapter

Unwind to when you were young.

I was fearful a lot when I was a child. And had the worst possible posture, slouching forward. My mom would constantly tell me to sit up straight and no matter what I did I couldn't sit up straight. It didn't feel natural. The startle reflex had already been ingrained into my body. But when I was active I was unstoppable and fearless. What a dichotomy. Timid in one part of my body and fearless in another.

MOVEMENT

DIAGONAL CRUNCH

A. Lie on your back, with your knees bent, and your right hand behind your head.

Inhale and arch your lower back, Exhale and while flattening your lower back lift your head and right elbow towards your left knee, inhale and lower the head and elbow.

Repeat 5 times.

B. Repeat the same movement with your left hand holding your left thigh underneath.

Focus on the sensations in your belly. Notice how the belly muscles lengthen when you, lower your head and elbow.

Lie in neutral. Pause, sense and feel. Notice your awareness.

Notice any peacefulness. Notice width, length, size, temperature, weight.

Notice any sensations of tingling or buzzing.

Notice any pain dissipating. Journal your feelings.

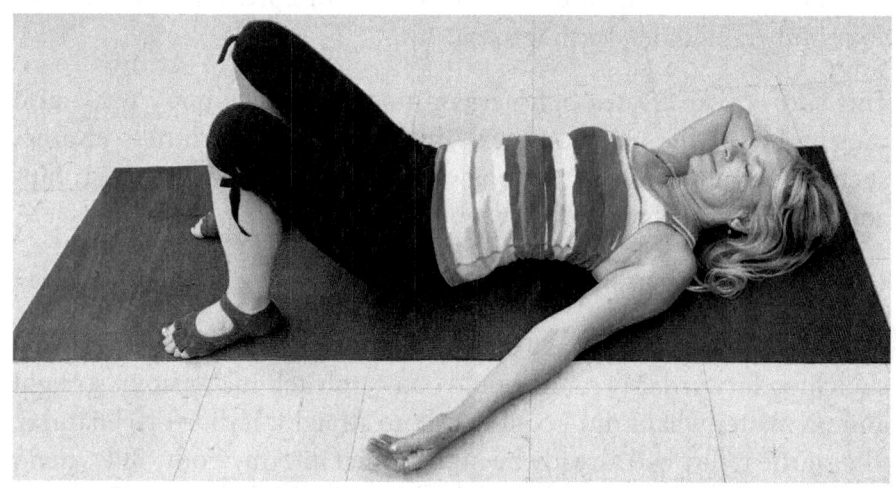

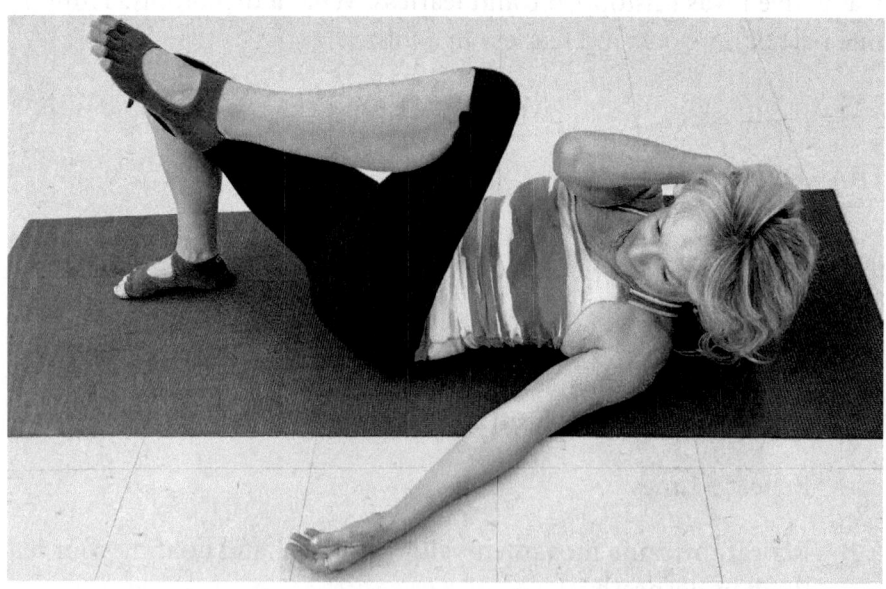

SECTION THREE

Releasing the muscles OF THE FRONT

SECTION THREE

Scouting the Barracks
OF THE FRONT

Releasing

Startle Reflex aka Red Light Reflex

ROUNDED POSTURE WITH A FORWARD HEAD

A habituated startle reflex causes all the flexor muscles in the body to tighten.

Things that may cause this posture to habituate: working at a computer, sitting for long periods of time, driving, whiplash, accidents, falls, sleeping in the fetal position, poor postural habits, low self-esteem, depression, fear, apprehension.

The startle reflex can be a reaction to fear. A balloon pops in front of your face, and you startle, automatically flexing the body to protect the center. This reflex is a normal reaction, but may become habituated in certain individuals. Fear may be of what others may think, fear of looking silly, or fear of being different from others.

Fear of falling is another fear that can be overcome by exercises found in The Divine Unwind.

Strengths: Abdominals and stomach muscles. This person may be able to do sit ups like they're going out of style.

Weakness: The back muscles may be very weak. Laying down on the stomach may be difficult.

DAY TEN

Emerge

*"See, I am doing a new thing. Now, it springs forth.
Do you not perceive it?*

The life ahead ~ What new thing is God birthing in you and then through you for others? It's time for that New Thing to emerge from the Spirit Transformation is never easy. It's not supposed to be. Let's look at the butterfly. They are lovely, graceful, as they flutter from flower to flower. But how did they get so strong and beautiful? How did they reach their destiny to fly?

Set your minds on things above, not on earthly things.

We know there's a transformation process called metamorphoses… The butterflies must move. They must twist in and out, stretch their bodies to strengthen their wings. This, alone, will enable them to fly!

First, we set our mind and heart on being a new creation. We have a choice to stop looking in at current problems, pain, worry, etc., and to stop looking back at past failures, disappointments, and things we were told we can't do….and to stop looking forward, worrying about the future with its feelings of fear and dread, and to start focusing on what we're becoming!! Being in the NOW, present with God.

"When going through transformation, focus on what you're becoming. Focus on where you're going to, not what you're going through.

In the unfolding, release fear, opening up to new possibilities, receiving healing, strength, and courage.

As you're unfolding, release everything that is not part of your destiny.

Kimberly Davis

Unwind to when you were young.

I was first aware of my peers at about age ten. Fear became my friend. It hung out with me everywhere. I was so afraid of being different than everyone else. I hid in a large suede Indian jacket. Sometimes, it gripped me. I began opening up much later in life after learning this beautiful movement, which exemplifies opening of the heart mind and muscles of the front of the body, erasing the effects of startle reflex.

MOVEMENT

BUTTERFLY

Just when the caterpillar thought the world was over… it became a butterfly.

Sense:

Lie in Neutral spine. Legs straight, arms at your side. Notice how you feel, the position of your arms (palms up, palms down), how you place your feet and legs. Notice the width of your back.

Rotate your head from side to side, notice any restriction in range of motion or pain or discomfort. Notice what you notice

Lie on your back, knees bent, feet together, arms at your side. Take a deep breath and as you exhale tuck your chin, lift your head up, look towards your belly, roll your arms inwardly. tighten your belly and squeeze your legs together. Take another breath at the top, roll back down, keep the chin down looking towards the belly, roll the hands outwardly, bring the knees apart. As you repeat this move work on coordinating the head, arms and legs to move at the same speed. focus on the sensations you feel while doing the movement and work on doing it smoothly.

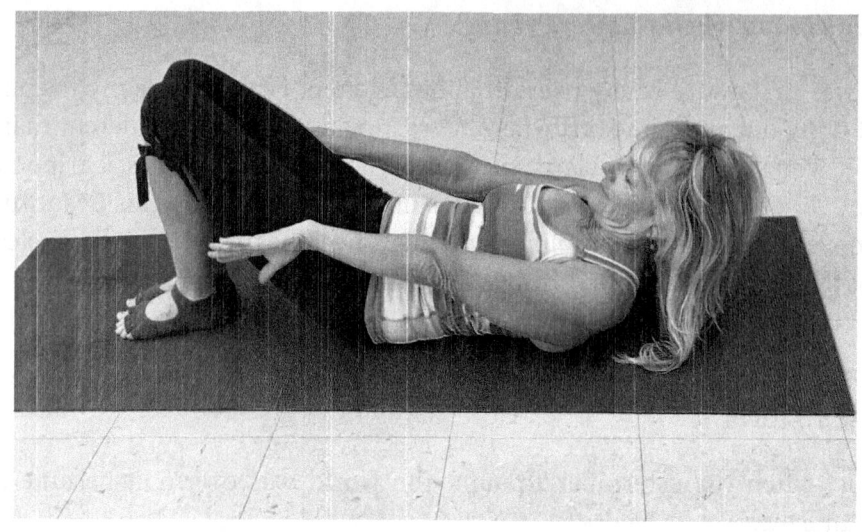

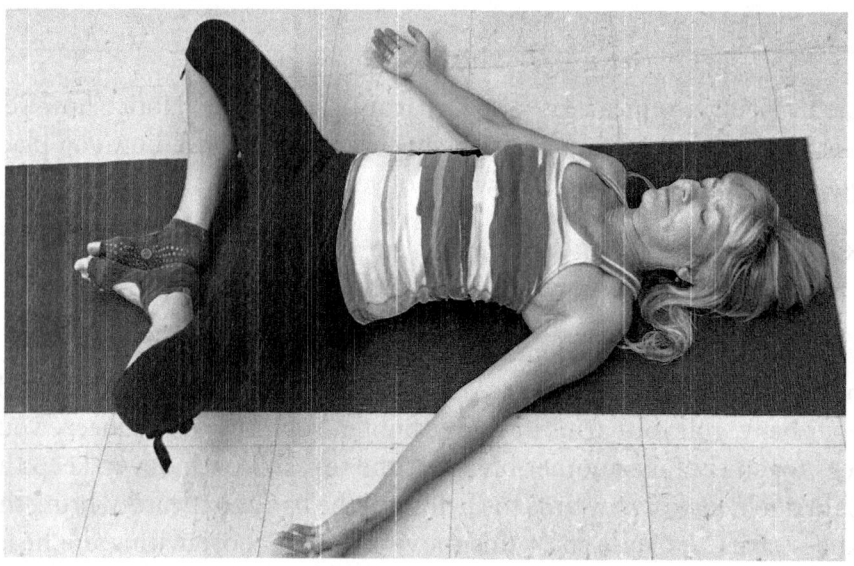

Sense:

Lie in neutral; sense the width of your back, sense the comfort of your low, back rotate your head and feel whether it moves better, smoother or has more range of motion. Notice when you ended with your palm up, did you roll them back down? End with the palms up.

DAY ELEVEN

Keep MOVING

Momentum affects every bit of you.

It's crucial to growth and getting things done. Like pushing a sledge down a snowy hill, creating momentum makes everything you want to accomplish with your divine unwind easier and quicker.

Newton's First Law of Motion — an object at rest stays at rest, and an object in motion stays in motion—is crazy important. Newton said that if you sit on the couch, you will stay on the couch. If you begin to move like a child, you won't stop.

It's a lot less work to keep moving once you have some momentum than it is to start moving from a dead stop.

By creating and riding on momentum, you will find it impossible to slow down. The more momentum you have, the more youthful enthusiasm you will feel. Your divine unwind will be unstoppable.

Your movements create momentum, and momentum creates results.

Do not dabble with your divine unwind. It requires focus, a decision to begin, a plan, action, and a continual commitment with little or no distractions.

Small distractions can have big consequences. Losing momentum slows progress. Don't underestimate even the smallest distractions. A simple phone call when you are beginning your movements can be a major diversion.

Every time you switch your focus to a new task or stop your movements to take in the distracting element, you lose a portion of that energy.

You lose momentum in the process. It takes even more energy to reach the same level of attentiveness and intellectual capacity you were using before.

That makes me tired even thinking about it.

Show up every day to your movement appointments, and you will build enough momentum to carry you back to your youth.

Unwind to when you were young.

One of my favorite things when I was young was rolling down a hill on my side. My brother and I would roll endlessly. This momentum exercise is actually a good way of balancing the body; just do it a little slower. Make sure you try both sides now.

MOVEMENT

CHEST OPENER

Lie on your belly

Put both hands under your forehead.

- A. Lift your head up and look up, put your forehead back down. Repeat 3 times.
- B. Lift your head and look over your right shoulder, lift your right leg simultaneously, lower and relax.
- C. Repeat on the other side.

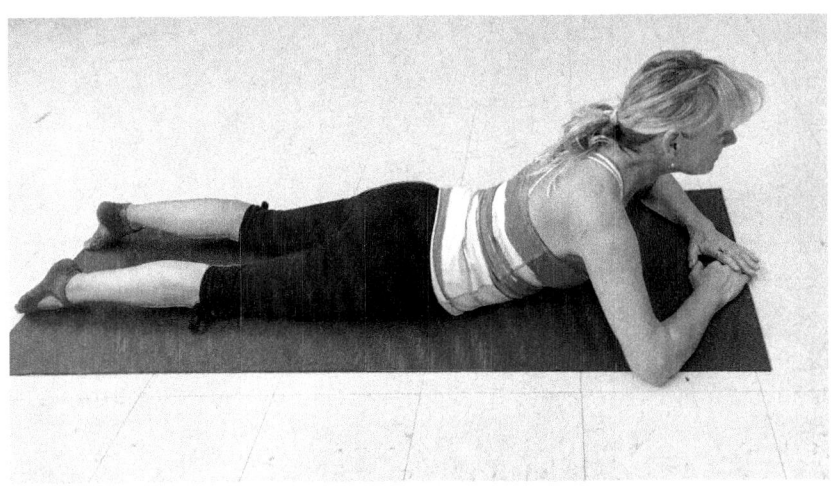

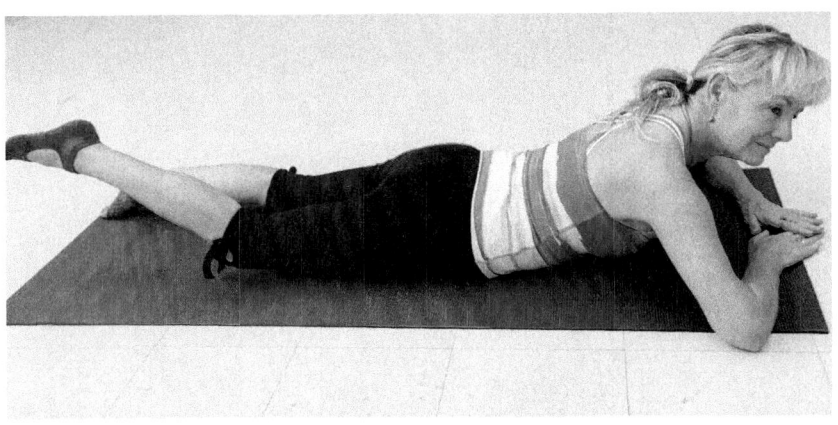

SECTION FOUR

Releasing muscles of the Waist
AND TRUNK ROTATION

Release

Trauma Reflex

A GUARDING OF MUSCLE GROUPS FROM A FALL, TRAUMA, OR SURGERY.

The shoulders may be at different heights. There usually is a dominant strong side and a rotation in the torso. This person may stand on one leg habitually or may lean when sitting or exercising.

Things that cause this posture to habituate: people who play rotational sports—such as tennis or golf—may get this posture. Standing on one leg dominantly, limping, or crossing your legs habitually. Twisting in one direction habitually or work-related repetitive-use injuries.

Strengths: One side is dominantly strong.

Weakness: The other side is very weak and may be atrophied.

Miracles are the ordinary stuff of God's day.

DAY TWELVE

Getting UNSTUCK

I work with clients every day who feel stuck. I tell them feeling stuck is an illusion. There is absolutely nothing surer than being able to get unstuck.

We spend most of our lives trying to decrease the amount of change we experience. We do everything possible to stabilize, routinize, and normalize.

We feel stuck not because we are actually being pinned to our lot in life by forces beyond our control. It's because the world around us whispered to us that the risks to get unstuck are just too great.

I know of captive baby elephants, who are sometimes chained to trees when they're young. As adults, they are freed from their bindings, but still spend their lives hovering around their home base.

The irony? As they mature, even just a bit, they possess the brute force to rip the tree out from its roots and free themselves. But they don't. They may have tried this when they were babies and failed, so the optics of the chains convince them they're still incapable of changing their circumstances.

The problem is not that we are stuck. It's that we become obsessed with familiar patterns, and that's what sabotages our lives and make us old and older every day.

When we finally reach the day when we're ready to change, we're up against a mountain of our own making. We have to untangle the deep associations that wreck our relationships. We have to face those fears, then choose otherwise. We have to admit that we haven't been as successful as we had once hoped before we can do more and become more.

And most importantly, we have to decide we want to stop the pain and discomfort that has plagued many of our lives for too long.

We have to unwind.

The cruel trick of life is that as long as we are like the baby elephant hovering near the tree we were once chained to, there will always be a gnawing sense that we have missed an opportunity.

Many will never commit to a divine unwind because it would mean exiting their comfort zone, and sometimes, it is the only one they have ever known.

But know this. You do not sabotage your life because you are stupid.

You do not sabotage your life because you don't know what you want.

You do not sabotage your life because you are incapable.

You sabotage your life when you become so used to your own familiar patterns, even though they are painful ones, that you fail to find the strength to endure the discomfort of breaking them.

Unstuck yourself and join me on the other side.

Unwind to when you were young.

I was never stuck. I loved all the messiness and unpredictably. I never enjoyed boundaries when I was a child. I loved the state of being unstuck.

MOVEMENT

SIDELYING

Sense: lie in neutral: Sense the left side of the body up and down several times. Notice the length, weight, awareness, or any discomfort. Sense the right and comare the two sides.

Lie on your left side, Hips stacked and shoulders stacked. Use your left arm like a pillow.

Modification; for shoulder pain or stiffness use a pillow. or bend your elbow

A. Hold the top of your head with your right hand, *Inhale* lift your head up side bending, notice the ribs coming closer together. *exhale* come down slowly and relax your head and foot. repeat five times.

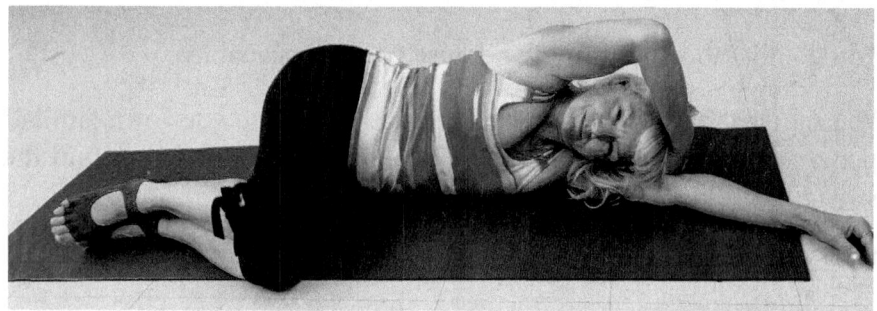

B. Lift your right foot up with the knees together *Exhale* and bring the foot down five times.

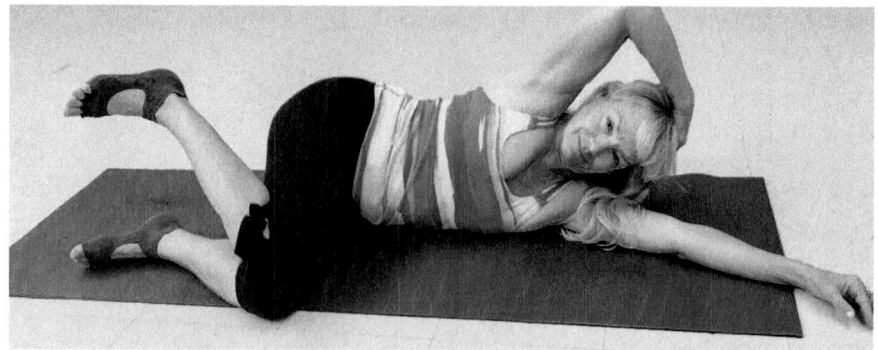

C. Lift your head and foot together slowly up and slowly down relaxing the head and foot each time. Your exhale should feel like a sigh. or ahhhhhh. Repeat five times.

D. Lift head and foot together, extent the arm and the leg out straight, lower the foot and hand down to tough the floor.

E. Grab your ear lobe and pull down gently while lifting your head, lower and relax repeat the next four movements on the same side of the body, then repeat on the other side of the body.

F. Clamshell

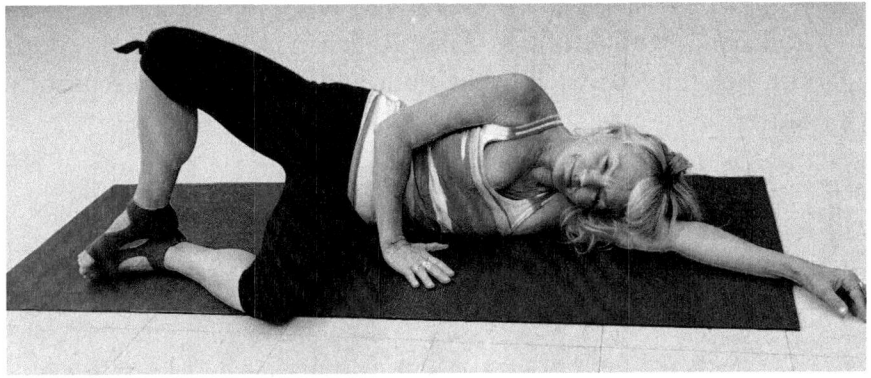

Bring knees apart and together super slow. repeat five times.

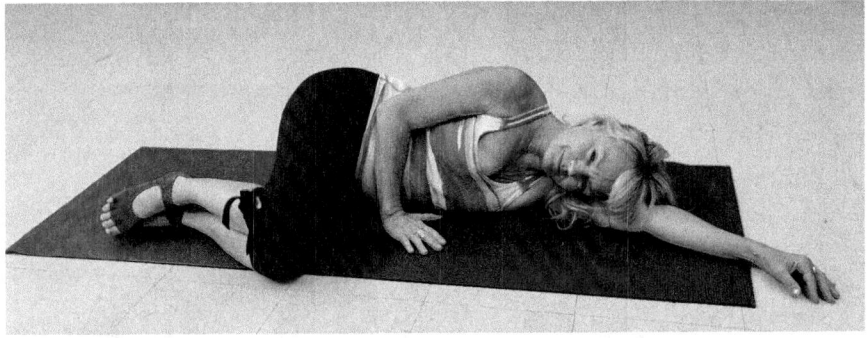

G. Rhomboid Arm Roll

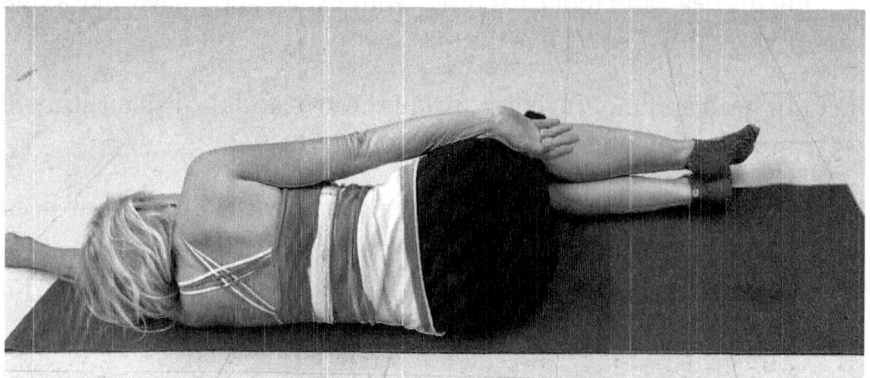

Roll arm in and out three times. Roll arm in, keep it in, lower the arm behind your back to the floor and back up again repeat five times.

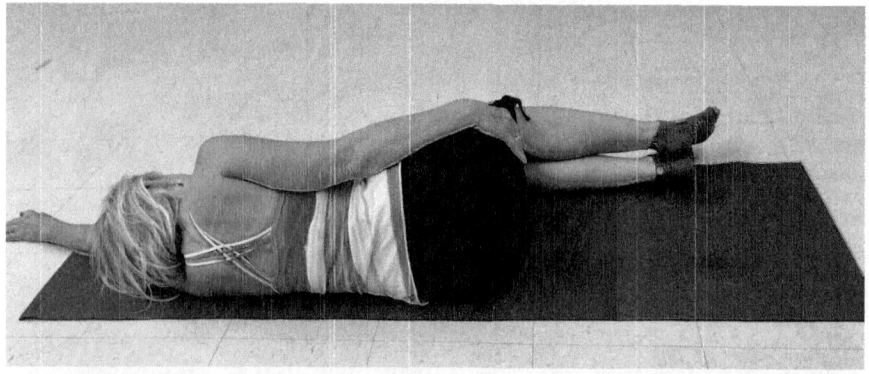

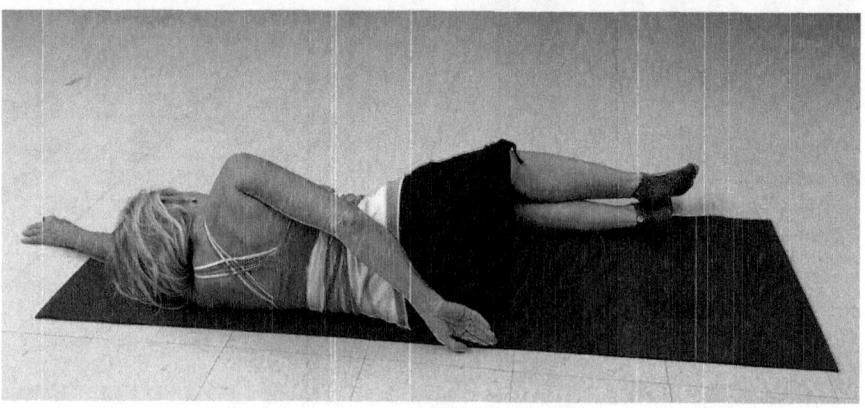

DAY THIRTEEN

What You Owe
YOUR CHILD, YOURSELF

One day, you may realize you are not the person you thought you'd become.

Maybe you thought you'd have bangs when you were a grown-up, or that you'd spend all your free time at the beach surfing. Maybe you thought you'd travel voraciously, or that your milestones would unfold seamlessly.

When you're young, you develop far-off ideas about what your life will be. Most of them aren't yours — instead, they come from the people around you: your parents' expectations, your hometown's cultural norms, and your friends and their values.

They're still shots from movies and magazines, images you conjured when you dreamt about what your life would be.

When you're young, you don't know enough about the world to make real decisions about who you're going to be within it.

One day, you grew up and broke your inner child's heart.

Looking back, you realize you've designed a life for a person that is someone else, not the person you are. You will learn the child in you grew up and got older, so old that you outgrew the dreams you had known.

What you owe that younger self of yours is a good life, a whole life, a pain-free life suited to who you actually are — a person you hadn't even conceived of. You can find inside of you the dancer, writer, builder, or artist.

What moves you?

What you owe them is the dignity and clarity to defend them, to heal them, to walk with them in mind.

What you owe them is not to cave to their youthful expectations, but to show them what's better, what's out there, what they're really capable of.

What you owe them is to fight off the diminishment of your body's resources and to reconnect with the vitality of your youth.

You owe them the best effort you have to unwind your life and celebrate the movements that you have known for years.

You don't need to be the biggest or the best. You don't need to reach the highest possible measure of success. Your job now is to determine how to best live out your truth, and to give what you are here and now to offer the world.

Your child is still in there. How magical, to show your child self that your dream was more possible than you ever knew.

From the Persian Poet, ♥ Rumi

We rarely hear the inward music,
but we are all dancing to it, nevertheless.
When the ocean surges,
don't let me just hear it.
Let it splash inside my chest."

Unwind to when you were young.

I think I learned how to dance before I learned to walk. From ballet at five to tap at eight years old and jazz in my twenties. Swing in my thirties, NIA in my forties, and spirit groove in my fifties. Dancing will always be part of my life. The Divine Unwind Dance has been waiting to bloom for a long time. I was born to do this.

What were you born for?

DENDRITES

The magic trees of the mind.

These microscopic tree-like branches grow on neurons in your brain when you do something new, like a new movement or learning a dance or instrument. Kids have a lot of dendritical growth with constant explorations of their bodies and the world around them. As we grow older and become more set in our ways or habitual in our patterns, the dendrites die off. This is how we get stiff, lose function, balance, coordination, and all the rest. Adults tend to have more habitual movement patterns which result in more stiffness and, eventually, pain. SOMATIC MOVEMENTS are magical in that they use the whole sensory-motor system, and adults begin to sprout dendritical growth, which makes you younger and also means they have more awareness available and a more intelligent system established in their body, muscles, tendons, ligaments, and joints.

USE IT OR LOSE IT

IT S MORE FUN TO MOVE LIKE A KID AGAIN

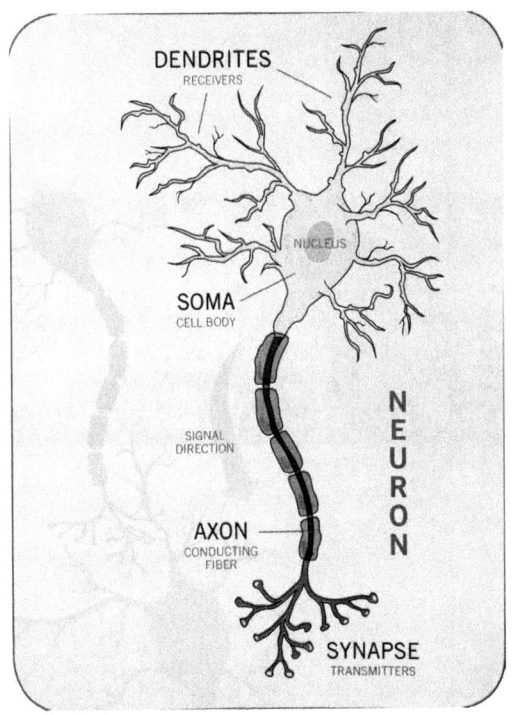

MOVEMENT

DANCER/RUNNER

Imagine your lying on a single bed. reach foreward to the corner of the bed with your hand, reach back with the leg to the back corner of the bed making a straight line diagonally, retract the elbow and knee bending a little roll your upper back onto the bed as you reach behind with the arm and reach the leg forward to the opposite side. reach back and forth several times slowly as if leaping or running in slow motion with one side of the body.

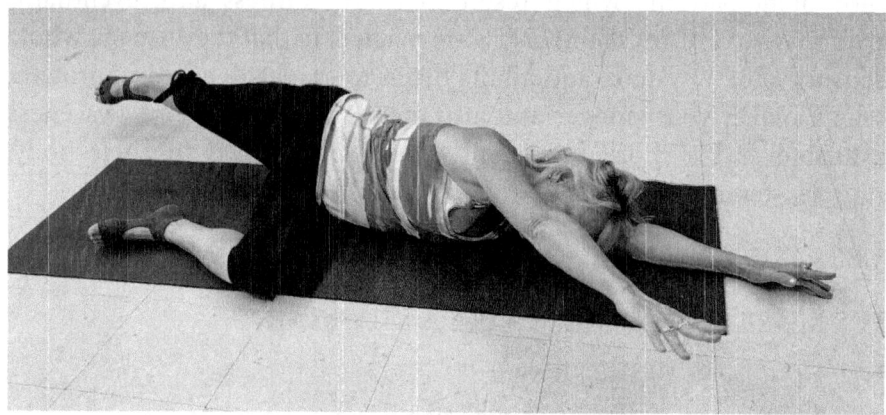

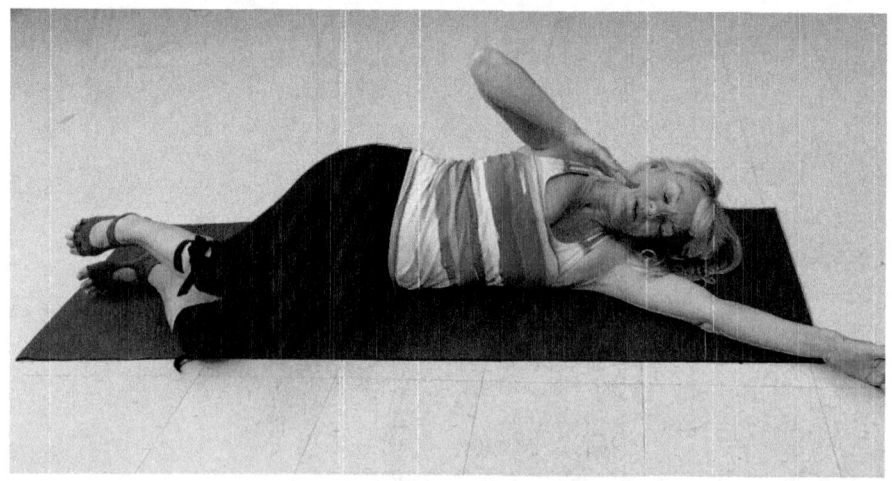

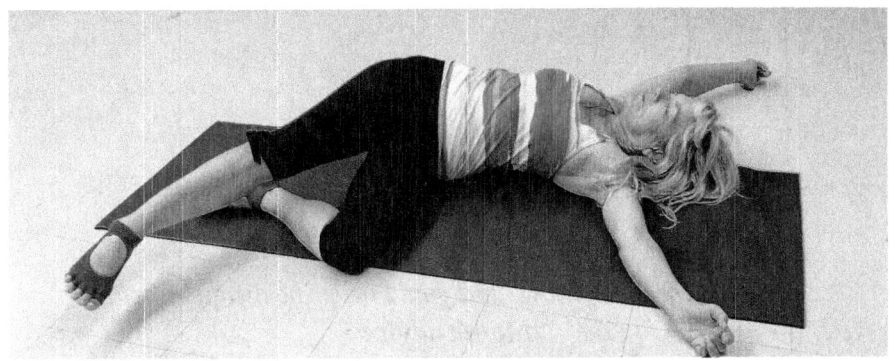

You are reeducating the walking pattern into the soma (living body) for smoother more effortless walking.

Modification; If you have hip pain either keep your foot lower and bend your knee more, or stop altogether and rest and skip the next move as it is an advanced version of this.

This movement is to release the strong oblique muscles on the side of the body, not the hips. go on to release the hips later in the book

DAY FOURTEEN

Expectation

"Don't expect anything, and you'll never be disappointed."
Mom's advice

There's a quote often misattributed to Shakespeare:
"Expectation is the root of all heartache."

Disappointment is inherently tied to expectations, and isn't something that can be washed away with a mantra or a little gratitude.

It's painful on a human level.

I have learned much about disappointment and about my own sacred journey. Disappointment is a reminder that there are varying levels to the human condition, that life is not just extremely high highs or low lows, but an ever-changing wave of emotional experiences.

They are proof that a rich, satisfying life exists in contradictions and shades of gray. Someone who experiences severe pain in their right thigh is capable of mind-boggling accomplishments. Another whose life has been rearranged by an automobile accident finds unspeakable joy with a loving family.

My family has taught me that sometimes, disappointment is a necessary ingredient for a satisfying life.

A life without disappointment is a life without expectation, hope, lofty ideas, and goals that make you uncomfortable. It's a life without growth. No matter how frustrated life makes us, our disappointments are indications of our sense of possibility. Together, we are able to rise above and beyond.

Its why I have given my life to lead so many back to their youth. Its inside the divine unwind, where disappointments become possibilities and all things become new.

Unwind to when you were young.

I remember being disappointed many times when I was a child, especially when I didn't get my way. When I was young, I would cry. I still cry. It makes me feel better.

I think disappointment is better served with tears.

It gives some relief.

MOVEMENT

COMPASS

In this version the arm and leg stay straight like a stick or propeller when the arm goes forward an inch the leg goes back an inch. Increase the range of motion as big as is comfortable for you. As your arm goes behind you the upper back comes down as well.

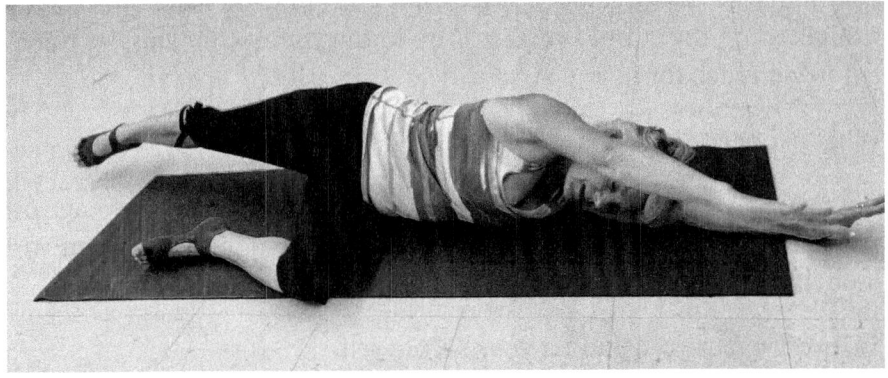

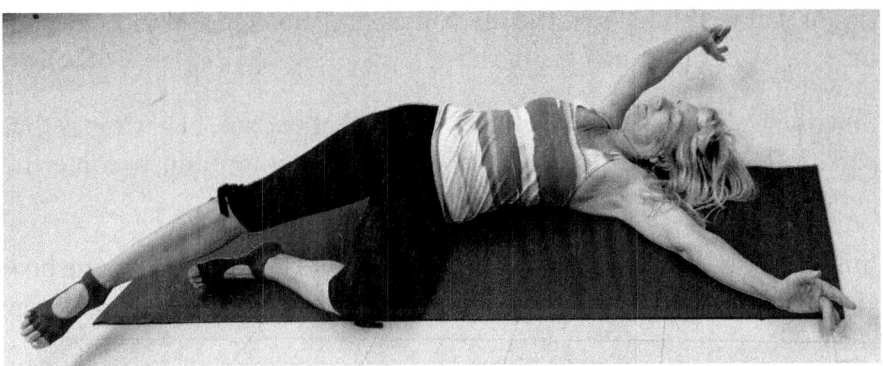

DAY FIFTEEN

More Out of
YOU

*I don't want you satisfied. With anything.
I want more out of you than you may want out of yourself.*

You know you deserve the promotion, but don't ask to be considered. You're bothered by being out of shape, but mess up attempts to work out. You want to dress well, but when it comes time to getting ready, you grab the same old clothes and call them "good enough".

You want to live in organized spaces, but don't find the half hour of daily straightening that would require. You know you need a glass of water, but never reach for it.

What happened?

When you were a kid, you were fearless. You reached for what you wanted, you stayed present, and you were more honest than you will probably ever again be in your life. Not much was good enough.

So, now, you are unwinding your sacred self.

I want you to think about the life you want. Pain-free and mobile, with the vitality of one much younger.

Imagine walking as that person, living as that person, behaving as that person. Every day of the rest of your life, wake up and become the person you want to be, full of life and pain-free.

Imagine how you will dress, how you will style your hair. Imagine how you write emails, how you handle conflict, what you get done, and how you do it.

Imagine your whole, full and unwinding self, and then, figure out how that person would handle the minutiae of your life.

Defy your old impulses. Refuse to stay small.

"Not good enough" will not be comfortable, but it is essential. You are not only capable of becoming this person, you are meant to *be* this person. Inside of your divine unwind, rewrite your story.

Unwind to when you were young.

I don't remember ever thinking there was something I could not do. I believed I could do anything I put my mind to. I was never satisfied. Ever.

I remember playing house and building forts and riding bicycles and kicking balls. I always wore at least one Band-Aid. I thought that was what work was.

MOVEMENT

HUMAN X

Lie on your back with your legs out straight apart in a V shape, and your arms overhead in a V shape.

- A. Hip Hikes; Hike your right hip closer to your shoulder lengthening your left leg. Hike your left hip up closer to your shoulder lengthening your right leg. Alternate, imagine waging your tail.
- B. Arms; Alternate reaching the arms using your waist muscles.
- C. Figure Eights; Alternate reaching with your right hand, left leg, right leg, left hand.

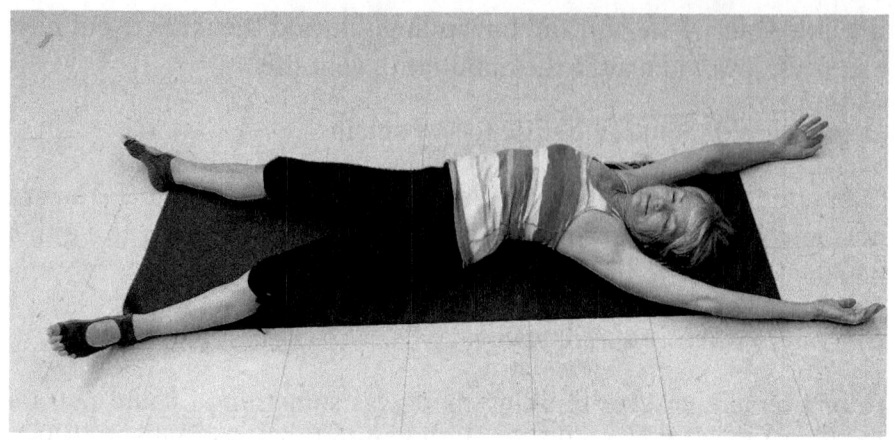

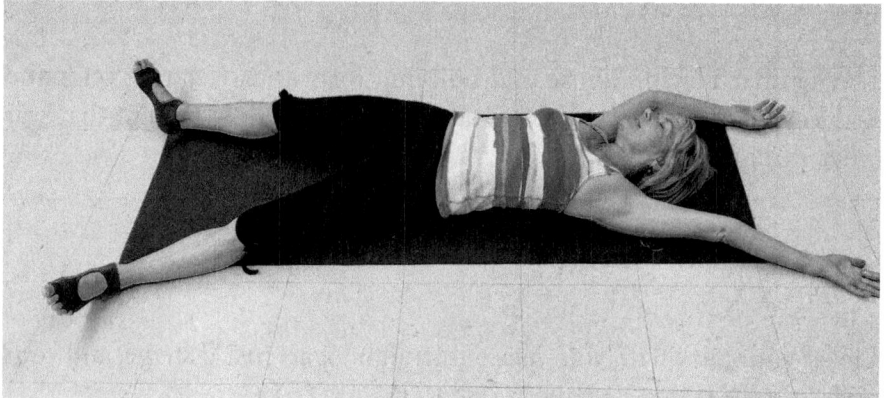

Straining and stretching do not work. Remember if you want to untie a knot, if you pull on it it will only get tighter. You have to gently undo the knot. Thomas Hanna

Modification; If you have a challenging shoulder keep the arms more down by your sides. work the arms in a reaching fashion slowly higher and higher. (Arms stay relaxed on the floor) Always work within your comfort level. KISS any pain and back off by bending the elbow a little.

DAY SIXTEEN

Meditation on a MEDIOCRE LIFE

There are many things you can do to unwind your life. There are also things you can do that will derail your mind for the unwind.

Make these mistakes for too long, and you become locked inside the garden of mediocrity.

At times, I have been there myself. Come into my office. I'll show you where the dragons are hiding to devour your divine unwind.

DRAGON #1: *Letting Others Dictate How to Live Your Life*

If you have certain ambitions, goals, and passions, pursue them, regardless of what other people think. Take control of your own life. Even though it may feel like it, no one can dictate how you should live your life unless you allow them.

The divine unwind and the road to a pain-free life isn't easy. Don't let others discourage you from what you feel is right.

DRAGON #2: *Giving Up at the First Signs of Resistance*

Some client begin the divine unwind and give up at the first sign of resistance. If results don't come immediately, they throw in the towel and claim that "it doesn't work." They touched the potential of an extraordinary, pain-free life, but, unfortunately, slipped back into mediocrity.

Not only expect the commitment to the divine unwind to be hard, embrace that its hard.

DRAGON #3: *Letting Fear Control Your Decisions*

Fear can destroy an intention within seconds.

But, as John Mayer said in his song, "The Heart of Life", "Fear is a friend who's misunderstood."

What if fear is actually excitement dressed up in a different outfit than we're used to?

Fear is an indicator that you've got an opportunity to do something meaningful and memorable. Developing an unwind of youthful movements is life-changing. Don't be afraid to commit.

DRAGON #4: *Letting Distractions Derail Your Focus*

Distractions are annoying and can lead to a lifetime of pain and frustration.

When you regularly let yourself get distracted, there is no meaningful progress. Micro-distractions are the most common form of distractions. Don't let email notifications, social media, news websites, and instant messages hijack your focus.

Before you know it, you get sucked into a vortex of distractions and waste hours of valuable time that could've been spent unwinding.

DRAGON #5: *The Knowledge Junkie*

"Knowledge puffs up, while love builds up." *1 Corinthians 8 1:b*

Some of my clients arrive as knowledge junkies. They know more about my work than I do and have never done anything about what they know. Consuming self-healing content can become a goal in itself, instead of serving as a means to an end.

DRAGON #6: *Allowing Yourself to Do It Later*

Procrastination is the mortal enemy of the divine unwind. We tell ourselves "I'll do it later," but later turns into "never" more than we'd like to admit.

It's the action takers who unwind their way back to their youth, not the ones who allow themselves to "do it later".

DRAGON #8: *Starting Your Day Reactively Instead of Proactively*

One of the reasons why many people stay old and hang on to all their aches and pains is that they start the majority of their days by underperforming.

They start it reactively by checking their phone or social media, immediately being influenced by the thoughts and agenda of other people.

They start it hurried and stressed, instead of calm and focused.

They start it by eating an unhealthy breakfast that causes them to feel sluggish and tired.

They feed their mind with distractive and mindless entertainment, instead of high-quality information that sparks new ideas and motivation.

You might have serious ambitions about the divine unwind, but if you start the day unmotivated, unproductive, and reactive to distractions and other people's requests, you'll have an incredibly hard time turning the rest of the day into productive movement.

Unwind to when you were young.

When I was young, I thought I heard a dragon in my closet. The next morning, I asked my mama if she thought there was a dragon hiding in there, and she said no. I smiled, much happier. But later, I thought, but what if WAS a dragon?

There are three large angels behind every dragon.

MOVEMENT

WASHRAG

Lie on your back with knees bent and extend your arms out in a T shape.

Roll your arms in opposite directions looking at the hand that is rolling upward, feel your wrist, elbow and shoulder rolling in opposite directions like wringing out a washrag. The knees are going towards the hand that is rolling downward. Notice how the spine is twisting in opposite directions from the head to the tailbone like wringing out a washrag.

Move gently with your body to gently unwind the tight muscles. Think of being lazy like.

Don't muscle it. Relax while moving and breathe deeply.

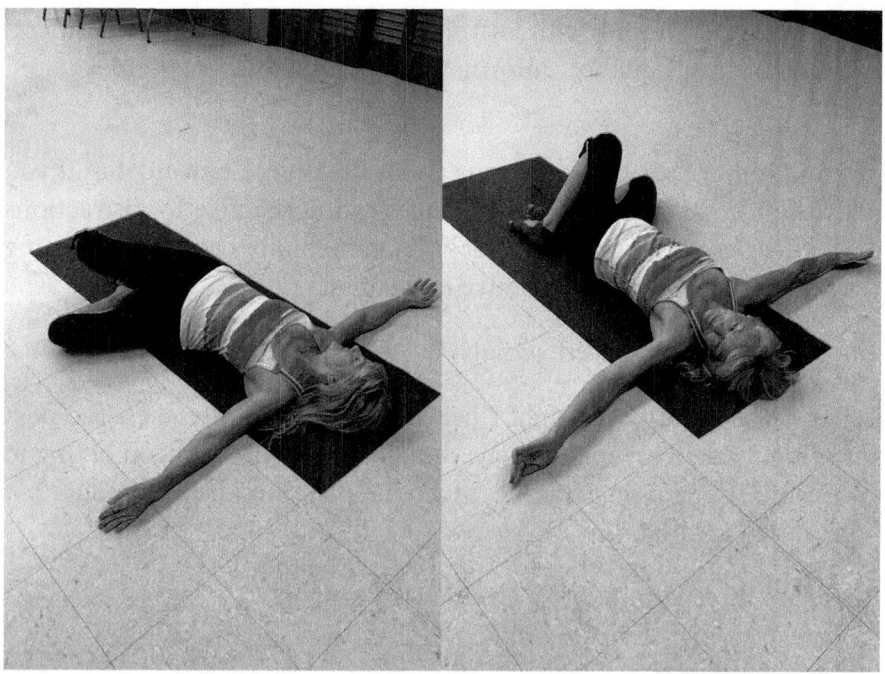

DAY SEVENTEEN

Shallow AND DEEP

If you wake up in the morning believing you have something new to learn, you will.

Some people dive deeper in their life than others, but everyone has the capacity to learn. Some will become involved casually with somatic movements.

Others are beginning a journey that will never end. They will become masters of their movements and their divine unwind will redefine their life.

Friends one day will say, "At eighty-four, she is the youngest person I know."

The ultimate aim of learning is to apply what you learn to what matters. Do you still remember many things and concepts you learned in high school or college? Hah. Probably not.

Most of what you learned in school had no immediate significance for your life and has been been forgotten.

There are two types of learning: shallow and deep. They are both useful for the divine unwind.

Shallow learning allows you to explore the surface of any topic. You accept facts and concepts with little or no reflection. It makes you a quick study on the thinking behind the divine unwind and somatic movement. The payoff is immediate.

If the topic is fascinating, and you want to walk away with a better understanding, you dig deeper. You move beyond the obvious, comparing yourself to who were yesterday.

Shallow learning leads to deep learning.

"Study hard at what interests you the most in the most undisciplined, irreverent, and original manner possible." — **Richard Feynmann**

For the deep learners, there is no end to learning about your body and soul as you divinely unwind.

Your brain has unlimited potential for learning

Unwind to when you were young.

When I was young, I skimmed over everything. I was so action-oriented that all I wanted to do was climb trees and run wild and free. I learned more from experience than I learned in the classroom. I learned numbers by playing Twister and memorization from song. I learned math by playing guitar.

MOVEMENT - CORKSCREW

Lying on your back with knees bent. Cross your right leg fully over your left leg.

A. . Inhale Lower knees to the left exhale lift them back up. Repeat 3-5 times.

B. Inhale Take the arms over to the right without bending your elbow or shifting the hands, exhale bring the arms back to center. Repeat 3-5 times.

C. Inhale Lower the arms first to the right and lower the knee to the left, exhale pull the belly in and bring them back to center. Repeat 3-5 times.

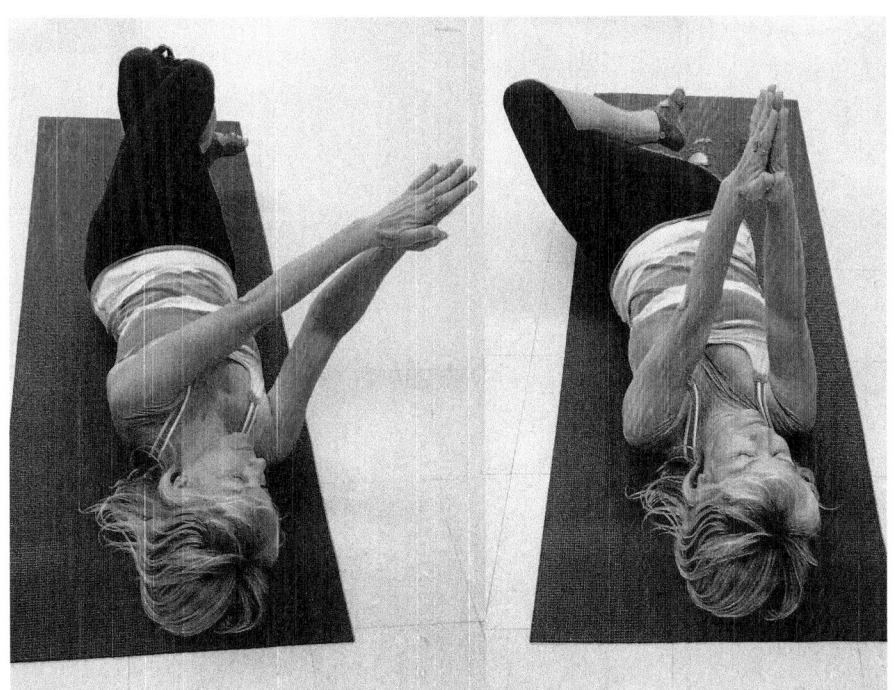

SECTION FIVE

Shoulders

Shoulder SECTION

If you have an old shoulder injury or surgery, masectomy, etc, this one can help unlock areas of disconnect, discomfort, and stiffness. Go slowly and KISS the pain and back off. If there is a segment that is difficult, gently, relaxingly roll into it. The more you relax, get heavy, and let go, the easier the movements become.

MORE CHATTER:

"My private muscle re-education has been helpful for me in managing chronic neck and upper back pain. The somatic movements are a toolkit, and I use them to tune up whatever area needs fixing that day or week. My muscle tension is due to prior surgery, but I feel less stress after releasing muscle contraction with the movements, and I realized a lot of my pain is my own creation! I'm aware of the way my body moves, the positions I stand and sit, and activities of my life that exacerbate and cause my pain, including the way I sleep!" **Dr. Karen Cadman**

DAY EIGHTEEN

A Perfectly
IMPERFECT YOU

Life is unpredictable. Certainly not perfect. But it's how we react to things that matter.

Your plans for tomorrow, next month, or next year may not unfold as you expect. So, what do you do? I love someone most of you have never heard of, Wabisabi, a Japanese philosopher who reminded me of accepting imperfections and making the most of life.

Wabisabi is translated as taking pleasure in the imperfect.

Wabisabi encourages us to focus on the blessings hiding in our daily lives, and celebrating the way things *are*, rather than how they *should* be.

It is a way of life that appreciates and accepts complexity, while at the same time valuing simplicity.

Thinking that runs counter to our modern world's relentless pursuit of perfection in possessions, relationships, and achievements.

Wabisabi is like thoughtful minimalism.

A common explanation is the example of a well-loved teacup, made by an artist's hands, cracked or chipped by constant use. Such traces celebrate that nothing is permanent—even fixed objects are subject to change.

Have you heard of kintsugi? Cracked pottery is filled with gold-dusted lacquer to show off the beauty of its age and the damage of the crack showcased.

Unbelievable. The fault is not hidden, but featured.

Wabisabi draws attention to the cracks in the teacup as part of the internal beauty of the object.

In the sacred scriptures, God is revealed as the potter, and we are the clay. Jeremiah 18 and Isaiah 64:8

In all we have discussed in Divine Unwind, nothing moves me as deeply as this truth of true beauty.

It is the language of the divine unwind, calling you you to relax, slow down, step back from the hectic modern world and find enjoyment and gratitude in everything you do.

I see you and I in all of our imperfections, our pain, our brokenness, and our damaged relationships. Our divine unwind treasures each crack in our portrait as reflections of our beautiful and evolving, youthful selves.

Put simply, the divine unwind gives you permission to be yourself. Embrace the perfection of being imperfectly you.

Unwind to when you were young.

Being German, my mom is a perfectionist. Our house and life was perfect—or so it seemed. Our house was so spotless I never had to clean. So now, I am very imperfect in all my messiness. I'm usually mad at myself for it. But today, I choose to forgive myself and find happiness in the mess.

MOVEMENT

ARCHER

The Archer is especially good if you have a challanging shoulder, old shoulder injury, surgery or chest surgery. It gently relaxes many muscles around the shoulder. go gently. If there is a particular area that is difficult work around the area don't push through it.

Sense; lying on your back in neutral spine. arms at your side. Sense the upper back. notice how the right shoulder blade feels and compare it with the left. Is one heavier or lighter? more aware less aware?, larger or smaller?

Lie on your back with knees bent, arms out stretched in a T shape.

A. Bring the right arm to the left arm and back 3 times. Allow the knees to roll to the left as you roll onto your left side.

B Touch the right hand to the right shoulder and then reach towards the left hand and past the left hand. retract a little bending the elbow and reach again rolling the hand downwardly, retract bending the elbow again and reach rolling the hand upwardly. Continue reaching in this fashion up a little higher towards the head exploring this section.

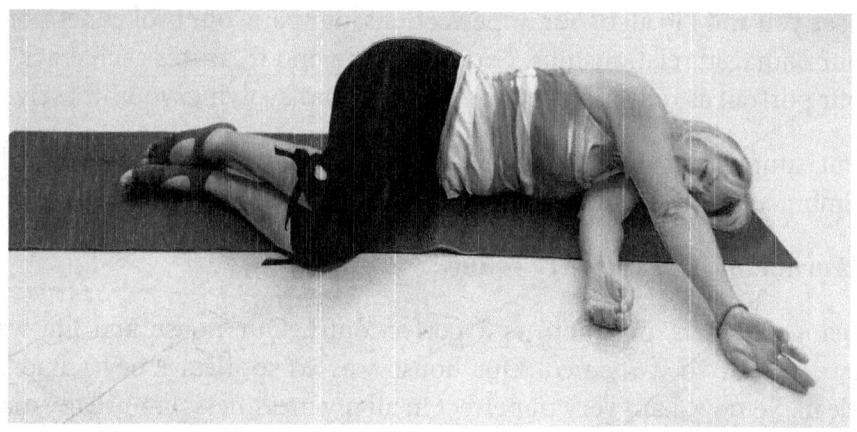

C. Bring the right arm back to the right you are back on your back again. begin reaching and rolling the hand up and down, reaching lower towards the feet inching your way downward.exloring this section.

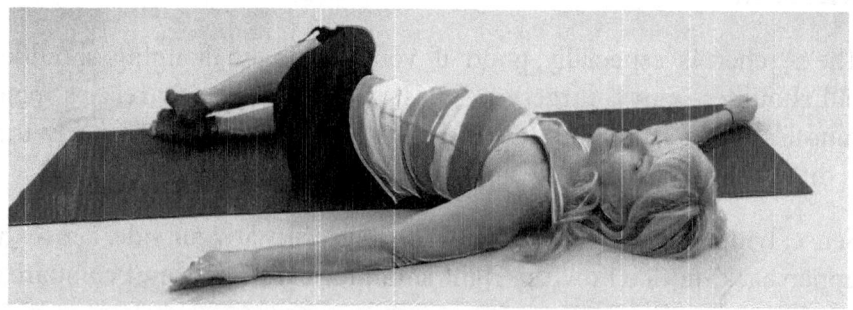

D. Bring the right hand back acoss to the left again, and begin reaching lower towards the feet rolling the hand up and down very lazily. (not stiffining the hand) and retracting and reaching, exploring this territory.

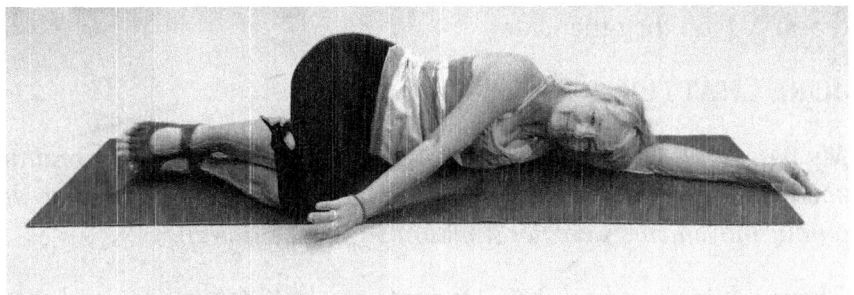

E. Bring the right hand back to the right and begin reaching higher headward little by little rolling the hand inwardly and outwardly

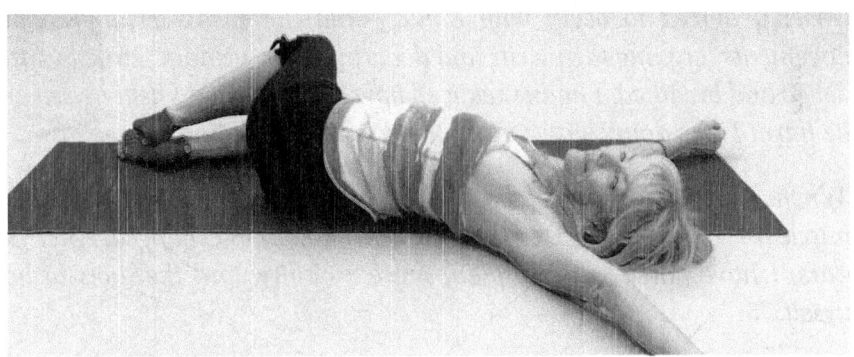

F. Be creative. You could go completely around in a big circle and then reverse,or you can just explore different parts of the circle.

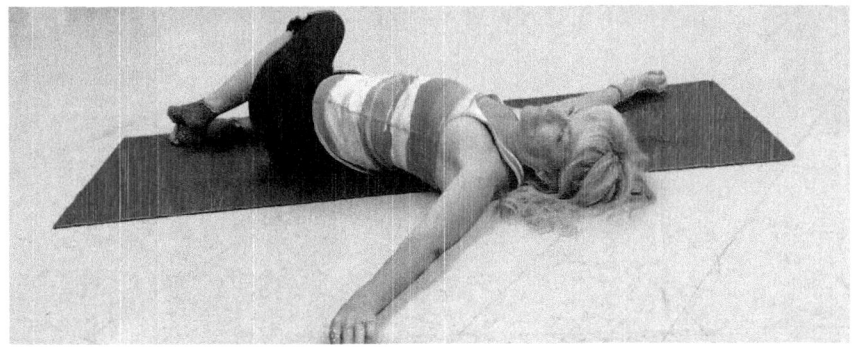

Sense; Lying in neutral again. notice how the right shoulder blade and upper back compare to the left side. Is the shoulder you worked with heavier or lighter ? more comfortable or less comfortable? larger or smaller? notice the awareness.

Repeat A-F on the other side

MORE CHATTER:

"My boss at work had watched my struggle with pain and the resulting mood and depression. She hounded me for months, explaining that somatic movements were not standard yoga-type training.

"I have a history of back pain, due to a congenital deformity and sports injury. My spine was fused from the L-5 to the sacrum. In 1993, I was victim of a botched surgery when the vertebrae above the fusion failed.

"When I agreed to begin with Linda Anna, I refused certain somatic movements, arguing the merits and debating their wisdom. Little by little, I let go and breathed. I hadn't realized how stiff and rigid I held myself and the harm I was doing with unconscious muscle guarding.

"When Linda encouraged me to lengthen and release my contracted muscleWs, I finally let go. In that moment, something changed. After two years, I have noticeably less pain, more mobility, and the tools to help myself.

"I do my movements every single day." **Claire Simon**

SECTION SIX

Hips AND LEGS

DAY NINETEEN

What I Would Teach
MY YOUNGER SELF

Most of what I learned when I was young, I learned from other kids. If an adult taught me something, the other kids had to vet it out before I could own it as true.

In my divine unwind, I have asked myself what I would want to teach my younger self as I meet her along the way. Here is what I would say:

Do what you think feels right. A lot of people have a lot of opinions about what is right. The more people you bring into the discussion, the less anyone agrees. Do what you think is right.

If you want a well-nourished body, order a lean meaty pasta with vegetable soup, instead of a greasy burger and fries.

If you want to go on a date with someone you like, for heaven's sake, ask. You have more to gain than to lose when you just do it.

Your health comes first, ALWAYS, ALWAYS, ALWAYS.

Take really good care of that body. You are going to need it, and the original tires and paint job is the best. A lot of people put bad stuff in their bodies. Don't do it.

Regret is more painful than failure. Failure only stings for a moment. Once you've learned what you did wrong and make the effort to make things right, that sting fades away. Regret, on the other hand, sticks with you for the rest of your life. So, if I had to make a choice, I'd rather fail a thousand times and succeed once than not try at all.

Be nice to everyone, even the mean people. Don't let others' behavior influence what yours should be. Kindness is stronger than meanness.

Stay in touch with people you care about. No one can stay sane alone. Never let someone you care about slip out of your life, even if they're living thousands of miles away.

Take care of yourself—you only have one you.

And remember the lady in the airplane's instructions. Put on your air mask first before your kids. Don't neglect yourself to fulfill other people's wishes.

It's okay to cry. For no reason. No reason crying is the best crying.

Let go of that awful moment that changed your life. It's not worth crying yourself to sleep every night for fifty years. These two words help a lot: "let go."

Money does not buy happiness. I can't tell you how stupid that is.

Become friends with a baby. Babies are the most magical creatures in the universe.

Give something of value to someone who has nothing. Then, look them in the eye and talk to them. Touch their hand, and say something nice about them. It makes you and the other someone more human.

Connect to a human spirit. Look someone in the eyes today and say, "I see you". We tried this at the somatic convention in Petaluma, California, and it changed me. I connected with people on a much deeper level, and I connected on a very deep level with my beautiful teacher, Eleanor Criswell-Hanna, the brains behind our work, whom I've known nineteen years, but not really that well.

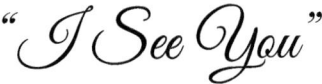

I first heard this term in the movie *Avatar*.

The aboriginal tribal girl would say this when she truly connected on a deep level. It moved me.

Younger self, I will see you on the way back in my divine unwind. You won't recognize me. I got old.

I will recognize you.

Unwind to when you were young.

I learned the golden rule when I was a kid,

and it stuck with me. Do unto others as you would have them do unto you. Jesus says it, too, in Matthew 22:37-39

"Love God with all your heart mind and soul, and love your neighbor as yourself."

These are the most important rules.

MOVEMENT

MARIONETTE LEGS

Lie on your back in neutral spine.

Sense; The left Hip, Knee and ankle. notice the length and weight of your leg.

Compare to the right. Notice any differences.

A. Tilt your right foot inwardly at the ankle and slide your right foot up towards your buttocks with your knee out to the right, lift your foot slightly upwards and inch or two, place it back down and bring your foot down to the floor and bring the leg out to straight. Repeat 3 times.

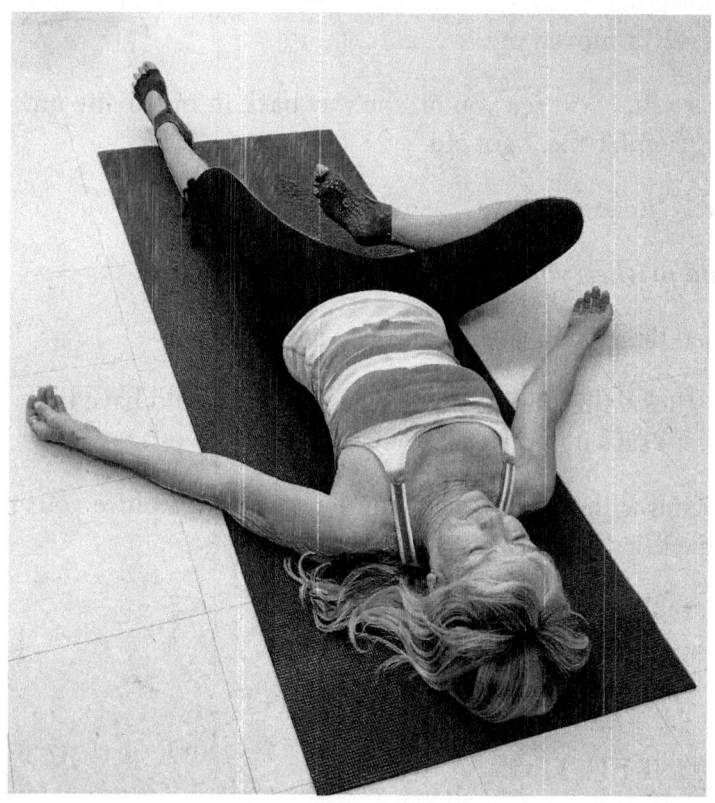

B. Tilt your foot outwardly and slide your foot out to the right and draw the knee up towards the left shoulder, lift the foot up off the floor an inch or two tilting the ankle, lower the foot and slide the leg back out straight. Repeat 3 times (knock kneed)

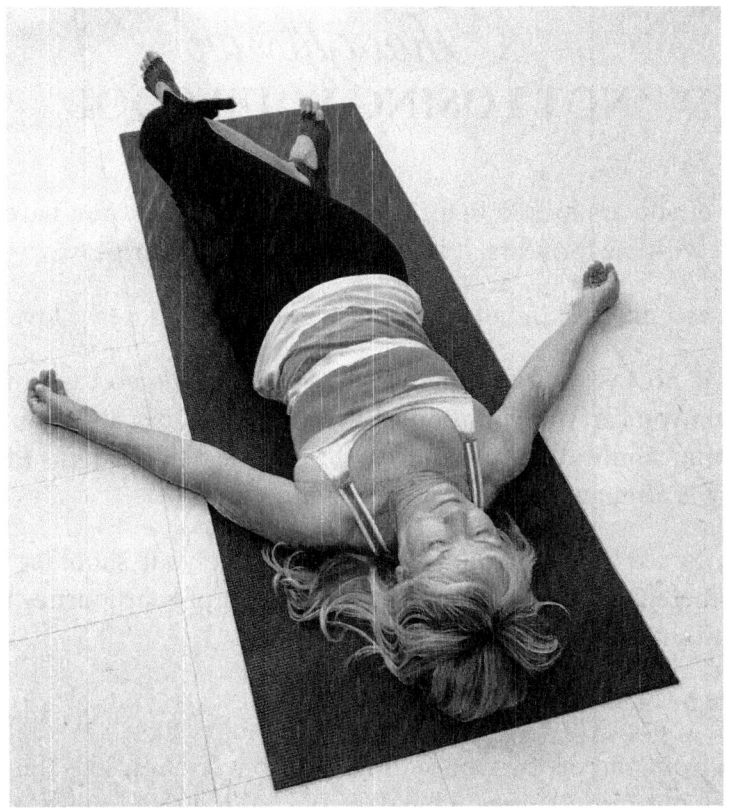

C. Alternate outwardly and inwardly 3-6 times.

Sense; In neutral, sense the leg again and notice if it feels longer, heavier or more aware, or more relaxed.

DAY TWENTY

Thoughts on NOT LOSING YOUR COOL

Some of you are locked in a titanic battle with anger. You have shared stories with me for years. It is a beast of a different stripe.

It causes a unique kind of pain as well as injuring those we love.

There is no easy answer to anger, just like there is no easy answer to the pain you carry in your body. In your unwind, pay attention to your returning youthful energy, and see if there are new thoughts that open up to you about where the anger is coming from.

Listen to see how the young you is hurt. Like your shoulder or your knee, there may be some damage to some part of your journey that can be unwound.

Or maybe blessed—yes, blessed.

Learn from the people you've hurt. A conversation like this can be painful, but it can help you bandage old wounds, and cause you to be thoughtful before you cause new ones. Forgiveness is difficult, but an antidote to healing on many levels.

It's quite okay to ask for help. You already know what it is like to live with pain, and you want to stop. That's why you came to me. Maybe it's time to stop this pain, too. They both hurt a lot.

Breathe, sweetie, breathe.

Unwind to when you were young.

I remember when I broke my wrist playing dodgeball in junior high. Everybody watched to see if I'd cry. I didn't right away, but a tear was welling up inside. The next day, I showed up with a cast up over my elbow, and a boy made fun of me. I socked him in the stomach, that was a gut reaction—somehow, anger came through. I never thought it through; it just happened. I've never hit anyone since. Sometimes, we don't know our own strength.

MOVEMENT

F.R.O.G. - *Fully Rely on God*

Sense; Lie in neutral spine. Sense the hips and leg muscles. Notice any discomfort.

A. With both your legs out straight and your feet together, slide both feet up with the knees apart, and slide them back down to straight. Repeat 3 times.

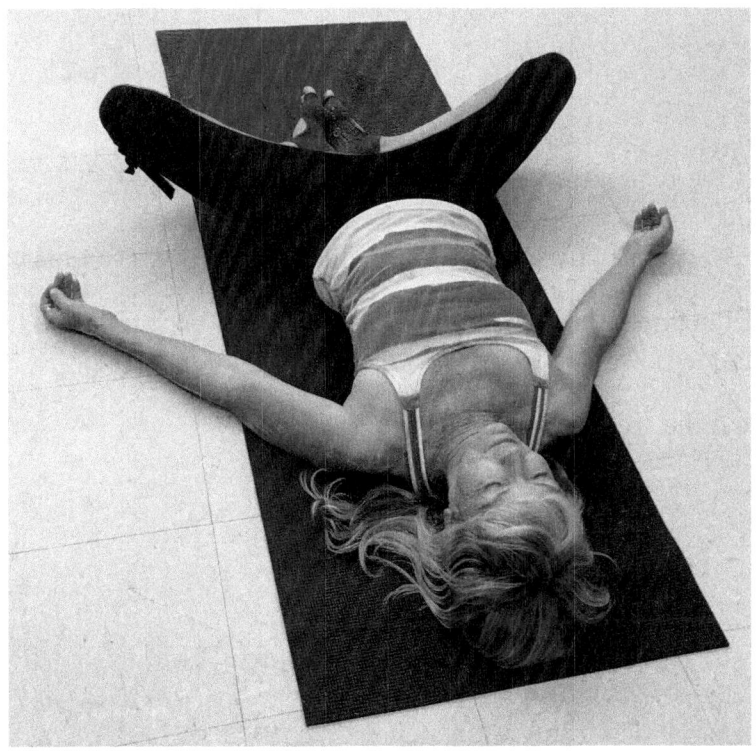

B. Bring knees together (knock kneed) and slide your feet up and apart, then slide your feet back down to straight. Repeat 3 times.

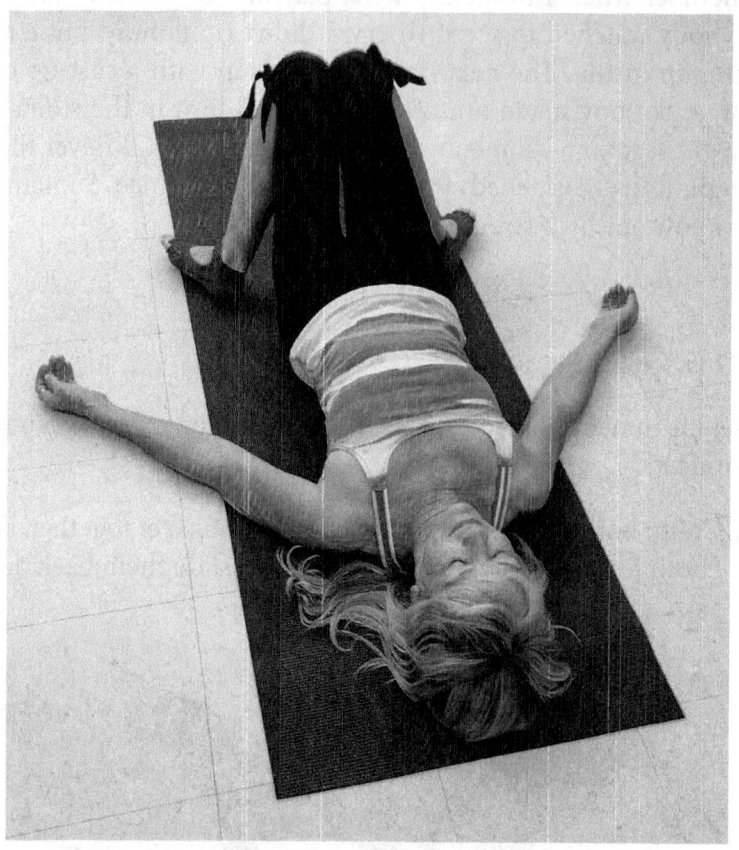

C. Alternate between the two frog like movements. 3-6 times.

Sense; Lie in neutral spine. Notice how the lower back feels and the hips and legs.

Notice if the arch in your back changes.

DAY TWENTY-ONE

The Art of SOLITUDE

> "All of humanity's problems stem from man's inability to sit quietly in a room alone." **Blaise Pascal**

> "All of humanity's problems can be summed up in two words. Put a muzzle on it" **Linda Anna**

According to Pascal, we fear the silence of existence, we dread the boredom of silence, and instead, we choose noise. We strain to outrun our emotions by the distraction of noise. In the process, we never learn the art of solitude.

Today, one hundred years later, Pascal's words ring true (as do mine). One word represents the progress made over the last century. Connectedness.

From the telephone to the radio to the TV to the Internet, we have found ways to bring us all closer together, enabling constant worldly and personal access.

You and I now live in a world where we're connected to everything except ourselves.

If Pascal's observation about our inability to sit quietly in a room by ourselves was true one hundred years ago, then the malady has become a worldwide pandemic.

Why be alone if you never have to?

The answer is that being alone is not the same thing as feeling alone. The less comfortable you are with solitude, the more likely it is that you won't know yourself.

Just because we can use the noise of the world to block out the discomfort of dealing with ourselves, that doesn't mean that the discomfort goes away.

Almost everybody thinks of themselves as self-aware. They think they know how they feel and what they want and what their problems are. But the truth is that very few people do.

In today's world, people can go their whole lives without truly digging beyond the surface masks they wear.

There is a solution. The only way to avoid being ruined by this fear, like any fear, is to face it. It's to let the boredom take you where it wants, so you can deal with whatever it is that is really going on with your sense of self.

That's when you'll hear yourself think, and possibly hear that still, small voice. That's when you'll learn to engage the parts of you that are masked by distraction.

The beauty of this is that, once you cross that initial barrier, you realize that being alone isn't so bad.

Boredom can provide its own stimulation. When you surround yourself with moments of solitude and stillness, you become intimately familiar with your environment in a way that forced stimulation doesn't allow.

The world becomes richer, the layers start to peel back, and you see things for what they really are, in all their wholeness, in all their contradictions, and in all their unfamiliarity.

Without knowing ourselves, it's almost impossible to find a healthy way to interact with the world around us. Without taking time to figure it out, we don't have a foundation to build the rest of our lives on.

Being alone and connecting inwardly is a skill nobody ever teaches us. That's ironic, because it's more important than most of the ones they *do* teach us.

Solitude may not be the solution to everything, but it certainly is a part of the start in your divine unwind.

Unwind to when you were young.

I used to spend a lot of time alone when I was smaller. I had toys I used to play with and used my imagination a lot. It was like I was talking to someone in my head, and it was me.

I don't talk to that person much anymore.

MOVEMENT

SNOW SKIIER

Sense; In neutral spine sense your hips, lower back and legs.

With your legs out straight, bring your feet together and pull your knees up to the left, then back out to straight. Now pull both knees to the right. Think about pulling your belly muscles in to drag your feet up. Alternate like a snow skiing motion. Repeat 6 times.

Sense; Go back to neutral spine and sense the lower back hips and legs.

If your lower back has discomfort after working on the hip muscles. You can incorporate a lower back release such as arch and flatten, arch and curl or diagonal crunch.

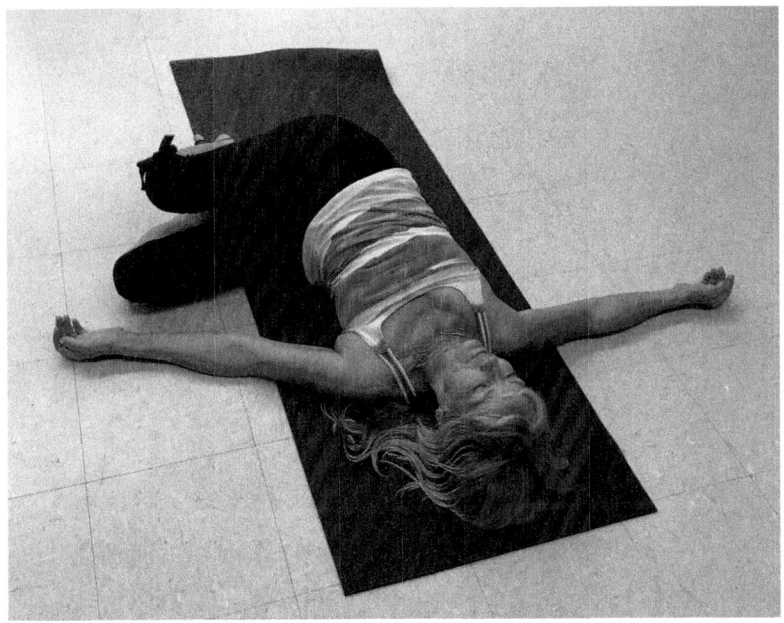

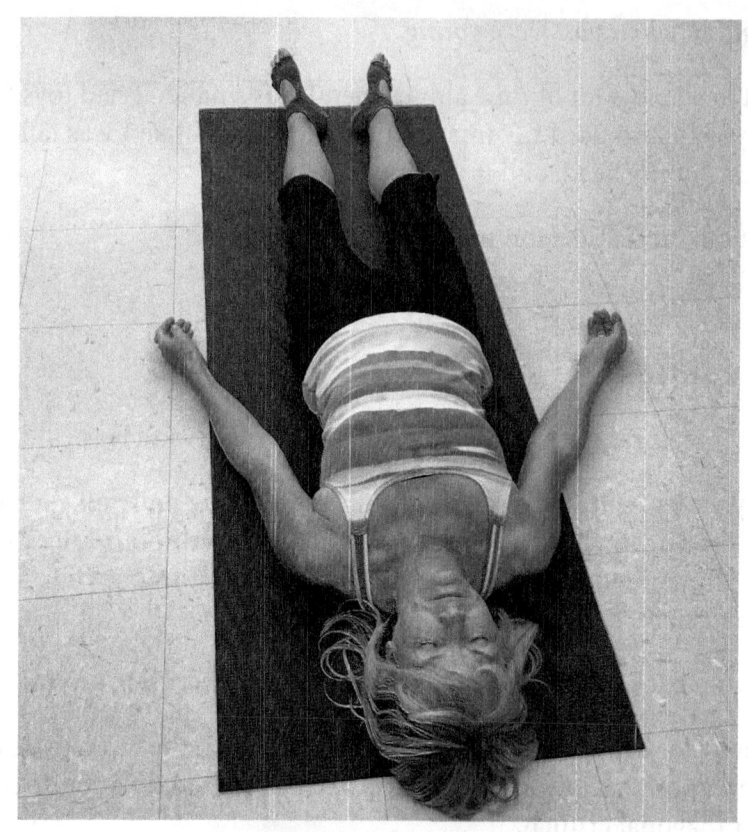

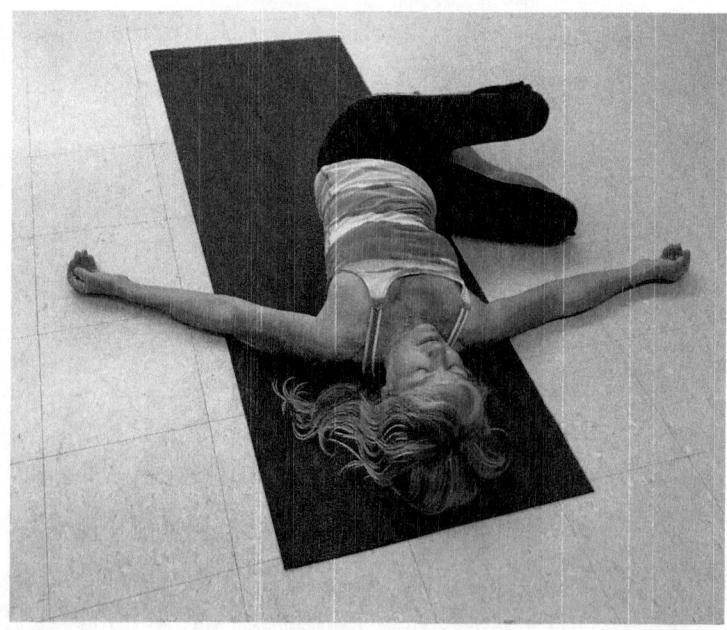

DAY TWENTY-TWO

No Bad DAYS

Sometimes, you just know. This is going to be a really bad day.

When you know you're facing down a bad day, it can feel as though the motivation has drained from your body. And when no one is around to push you, things you've committed to doing, things you want to do, can lose all appeal.

When you feel this happen.

You convince yourself that these things don't matter to anyone else, and shouldn't matter to you, either. You see an endless gray horizon of indifference, and think: "Nope, not today."

A fundamental mistake people make is believing that motivation is supposed to be there before you begin working on something, and if it's not, you probably shouldn't be doing that thing in the first place. Not feeling it today? Let's see what tomorrow looks like.

But that is not how our brains work. The motivation isn't there because your imagination is operating in reverse, filling in the gaps of a messy day with unmotivating options.

Someone once suggested on the bad days, we pull out the 'do-something' principle.

It's the idea that action isn't merely the effect of motivation, but also the cause of it. If you actually begin doing something that you are usually motivated to do, the something that you do will create momentum toward the thing you really want to do.

Your golden ticket to the divine unwind.

You will be so surprised at the results when you begin unwinding and trusting in the healing and letting go of whatever ailing you. The momentum of the movements and time spent in the sacred space will refresh your mind and body and spirit. I even do the movements when I'm sick and have felt 30% better after the movements.

And we know some days it won't be exciting to spend time with your movements, because you just won't want to. I want to suggest that you will fall in love with the movements; you did them when you were young, they are organic to our bodies. Your body needs it, and it will crave it after a while. For me, it took about two years before I craved the movements.

Unwind to when you were young.

I loved moving all the time when I was young. I skipped, jumped, skated, slid, and fell through most of my days. I enjoyed every moment of life. Especially the raindrops and snowflakes.

MOVEMENT

HAMSTRING CURL strap optional

Lying on your back with the strap under the ball of your foot. Or put your hand on the inside of your foot. Hold the foot lightly.

- A. Bend your knee to your chest, and extend your leg out straight. Flex your ankle. Continue bending and lengthening your leg upwards or put your left hand on the inside of your left foot (as in the picture) Repeat three times.

    Imagine you're shining a light out your heel.

- B. Take the leg to the right side of the body and do the same action.

- C. Take the leg to the left side of the body, bending and extending the leg.

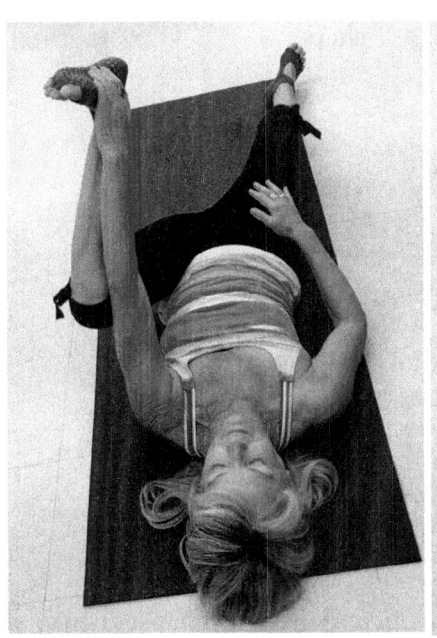
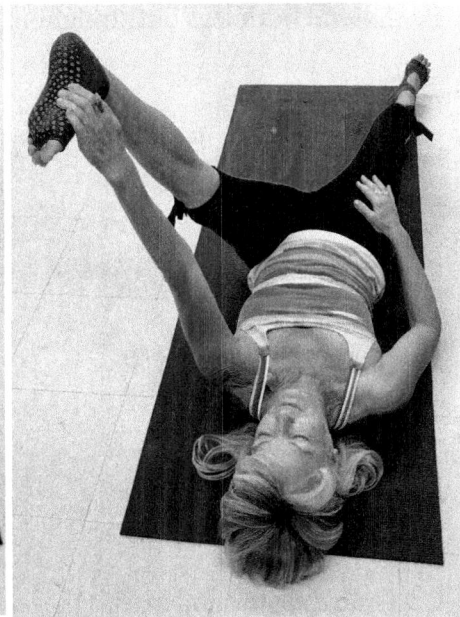

HAPPY BABY. Put the strap down

A. Bring your feet together, with your knees apart. Grab the inside of your feet, extend one foot out at a time towards the sky. Alternate.

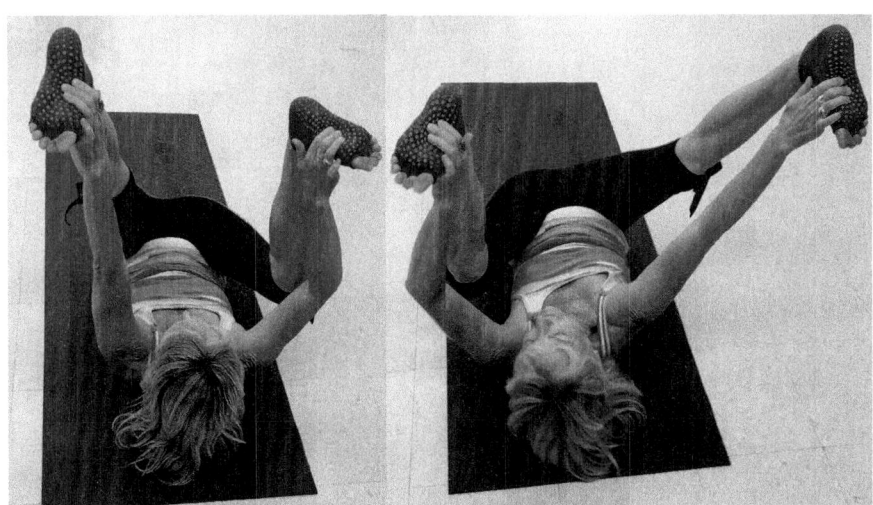

B. Extend both legs out straight in a V shape.

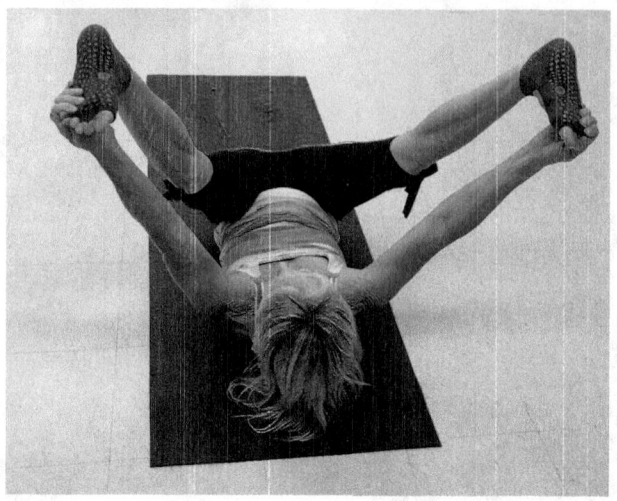

C. Grab each toe and extend the leg out and in. This synapses neurons in the feet.

Be creative, clap your feet together. ;)   I saw a new born doing all of these moves in a grocery store. She was so joyful and happy and finished with clapping her feet.

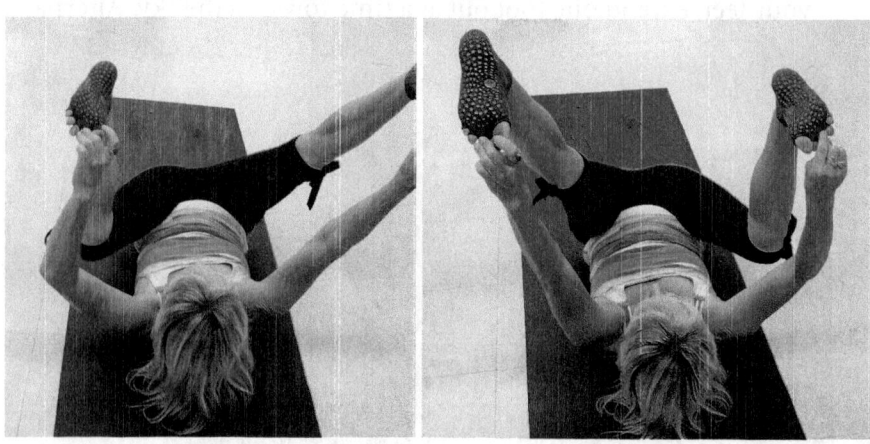

You're done. :)

DAY TWENTY-THREE

Mastering The DIVINE UNWIND

You are all on a journey of becoming.

A tree gives glory to God by being a tree. I contemplate the trees, and it reminds me to reach upwards to give thanks to God, who is higher and wiser than I.

In mastering the divine unwind, there is thinking that reliably and consistently leads to highly productive movements.

Principle #1: When You Choose to Move, Choose to Relax

Most people are never entirely on and never fully off.

When they're doing one thing, they are always doing another. Every few minutes, there are distractions, phone calls, television, and conversations. The boundaries between personal space and the outside world have disappeared. It is not helpful in the moments of unwinding.

Be intentional with your divine unwind. Be thoughtful and completely present. Turn off the distractions, go inside of your interior space, and lock the door.

Principle #2: Don't Dabble

Your divine unwind is essential to your life ahead.

In reality, only a few things in life truly matter. Only a few activities significantly move the needle towards unlocking your youth again. You must choose the vital among the trivial.

There are lots of things you can do that might help. There are few that matter.

Principle #3: Create Clarity on a Daily Basis

Procrastination hardly ever comes from laziness or a lack of motivation. Instead, it comes from not having enough clarity.

Many search for motivation when they are really looking to simply understand what they are to do.

Most people fail to create a clear plan for their day, which is why they stumble into the evening not having achieved anything they value.

They act impulsively and unfocused, instead of consciously following a clear path.

PAUSE; take a deep breath, uncross your legs. Check in with your thoughts. Take captive any thought that is negative. Imagine you have a catcher's mitt that you can catch any negative thought with. NOW, throw it away.

Look down at your feet. This is important, where you are right now, and where you are headed. Take a moment to reconnect to the Divine, coming into the present.

Don't lose your connection to your divine unwind inside the messiness of a cluttered day.

Sit down in the morning, write down your priorities, and make a "to do" list for the day every morning. It takes three minutes. Becoming clear about what matters for the day means becoming clear about what does not. If morning doesn't work for you, plan ahead in the evening.

Principle #4: Prioritize Your Divine Unwind

Your health is like a precious diamond, and you are in charge of it. To live a life of vitality, the somatic way is vital. Make it a priority. Think about how much time we waste going to do our nails, hair, and eyebrows. It's ridiculous how much money we spend on the external, but if you don't have your health, none of it matters. Stay strong. It's more fun.

Unwind to when you were young.

I always loved looking forward to something when I was a child. An upcoming birthday party, a visit to a friend's house. I loved the thrill of anticipation. It was like a drug.

Anticipation, anticipation is makin' me late, it's keepin' me waitin'…
Carly Simon

MOVEMENT

GLUTE CIRCLE

With knees bent, cross your right leg over your left leg, and lift the legs in the air. Draw a small circle in the air, slowly sensing and feeling the tush. Repeat in the opposite direction.

Repeat five to six times

Relax with legs out straight. Notice the difference between the left tush and the right. Sense the weight and comfort. Notice your low back.

Repeat on the other side.

Sense; lie in neutral, sense your right and left buttocks. Notice the weight. Notice any discomfort in the butt or low back.

Modification; you can put your hands behind your legs, or you can use a strap.

Sense; Notice the buttocks again. Is it more relaxed? Are you more comfortable?

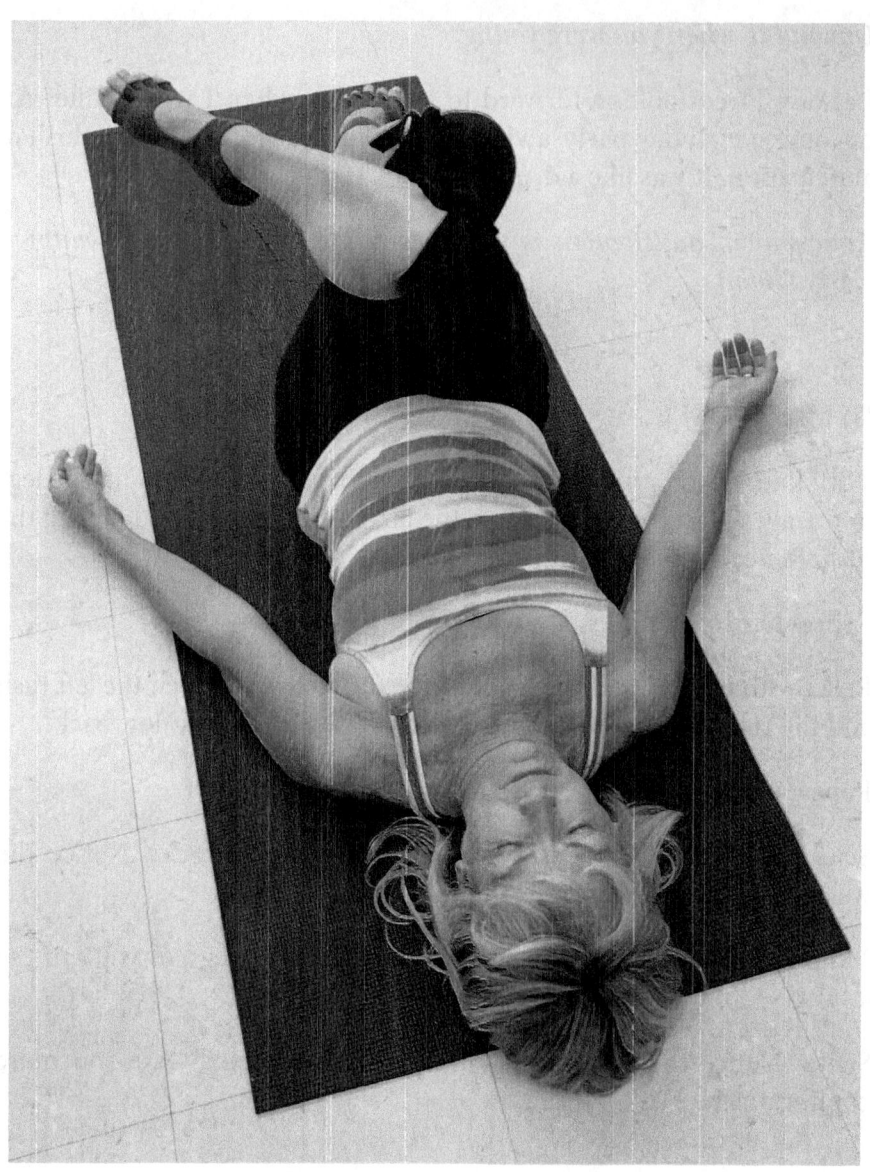

Why do I keep saying slow down? Your brain is sending messages back and forthto the muscles in a motor feedback loop. In order to get clear information about what your doing you must go slowly. If you speed up another part of the brain takes over and the brain gets cluttered information.

DAY TWENTY-FOUR

Two Secrets to the DIVINE UNWIND

There are a many moving pieces in considering a lifestyle change as suggested in Divine Unwind. There is not only understanding the thinking, but the movements, the scheduling, the progress, the strategies - a lot of stuff.

I felt the same way. Eventually, there came a moment when I realized that all the possibilities and reading and conversations were only stalling me from the real work of actually beginning my personal sacred journey into the unwind. I knew what I needed to know. It was just a matter of using it.

My youth was back there somewhere. I needed to go get it.

I found the two simple secrets for my divine unwind to become a reality. I needed to physically move my booty into position for my movements. Then, I needed to begin the simplest part of my first movement.

That's it. That's the whole thing. It's simple, but it isn't easy.

Oftentimes, we do everything in our power to avoid that first step. We grab another cup of coffee, go for a walk, read a book, run errands. I actually spent time rearranging my bookshelf before I wrote this, if you can believe it. I tried to escape. The voice inside my head told me to turn on Hallmark.

But instead, I laid down on the floor, I put my phone away, and I closed my internet browser. And I started doing a somatic movement from this chapter. Then, like magic, I was feeling good while doing it. And the bonus was the relief and comfort I felt after.

The real secret of this technique is that you must do it again tomorrow, and the next day, and the day after that. Build up momentum, and keep it.

I call it your One-A-Day Divine Unwind Vitamin. Just do one movement every day, and your divine unwind will explode.

We can talk about the great thinking and what happens all day, but doing so won't get the real work done. At some point, you have to just get started.

Unwind to when you were young.

I never remember overthinking anything when I was very young. If something made sense, I just did it. If anything, I could have used a bit more thinking ahead, rather than less.

MOVEMENT

GLUTE-PIRIFORMIS-CIRCLE

Cross your right ankle over your left knee, lift the legs up in the air. Apply a little pressure between the ankle and the thigh. Draw a circle with your legs. Go slowly

Modification; You can put your hands behind your legs or use a strap.

Place the left foot on the floor, arms extended out straight. Lower the right foot to the floor to the left, and lift back up again. Pull your belly button in to lift the legs back up.

Repeat 3 times.

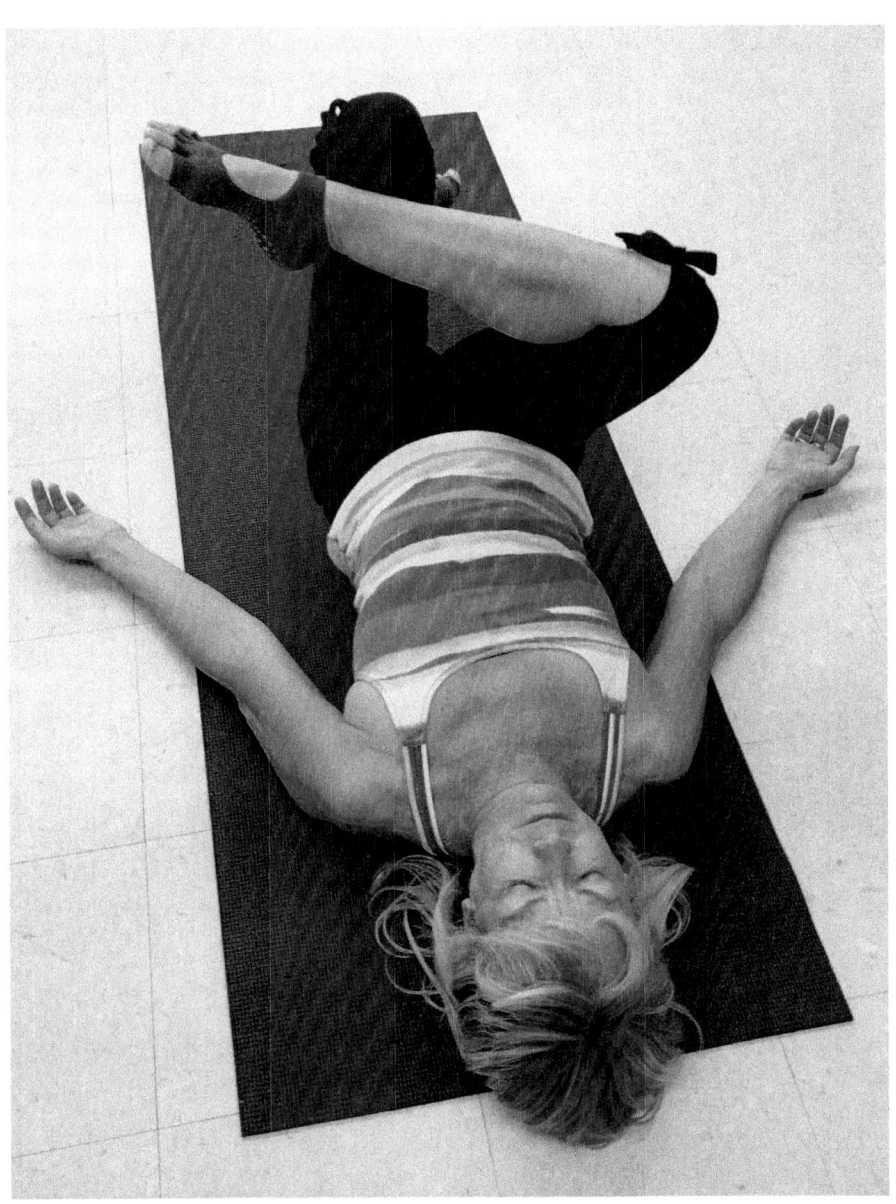

SECTION SEVEN

Neck and SHOULDERS

DAY TWENTY-FIVE

Thinking Younger
THROUGHOUT THE DAY

It's remarkable the effect the divine unwind will have on the rest of your day. Thinking about being young in your body affects your awareness of your sacred journey every few minutes. The youthful energy can become intoxicating.

The right hemisphere is your creative side. It knows how to do just about everything. It trusts and it's intelligent.

The left hemisphere is the analytical side. It likes to critique and tell you what to do. It's like having your best friend sitting next to you, criticizing you constantly. If you quiet the left side, the right side knows how to do it, balance, play, dance.

Start paying particular attention to your thoughts. Simply notice what you are thinking. You are beginning to think differently here and there, thoughts you may not have considered before. Opinions of others you may have judged before suddenly seem a bit more interesting.

"As a man thinks in his heart, so he is." **Proverbs 23**

If your body is becoming younger by your movements, expect your thinking to do the same.

Begin to live with your thoughts in the present moment. When you are doing something you actually like, no matter how big or small, genuinely enjoy it. When you are listening to music, watching a movie, or spending time with your family and friends, unwind into the moment as you did when you were young.

Don't think about goals, failures, or things you have to do tomorrow. Just be there. Right now. Just like the moment that you're taking to read these words. When it's gone, it's gone forever. Realize that on a deeper level, and you'll never even dare to leave the present.

It's where the divine unwind leads. We become younger and younger and younger until we find ourselves back in the present moment.

And we never, ever, leave it again.

Unwind to when you were young.

When I was a child, I was very much in the present. Every moment counted. I was touching bushes, twirling around, playing with my feet, and bouncing everywhere. I didn't worry; it wasn't in my vocabulary.

MOVEMENT

SPANISH DANCER

A. Sitting with your feet to the left and your knees to the right, place our left hand on your right shoulder and your right hand on the floor beside you. Rotate all the way to the right, Pause and take a picture of what you see. Rotate everything together to the left and right 3 times slowly and effortlessly, end to the right

B. Rotate the head only 3 times.

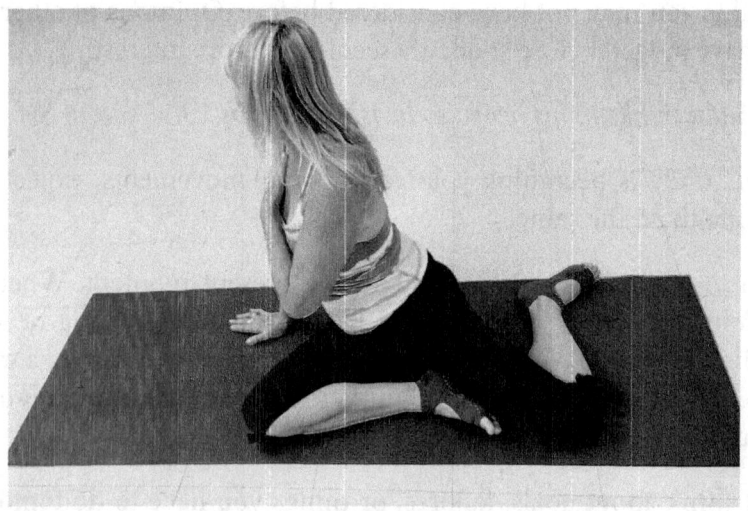

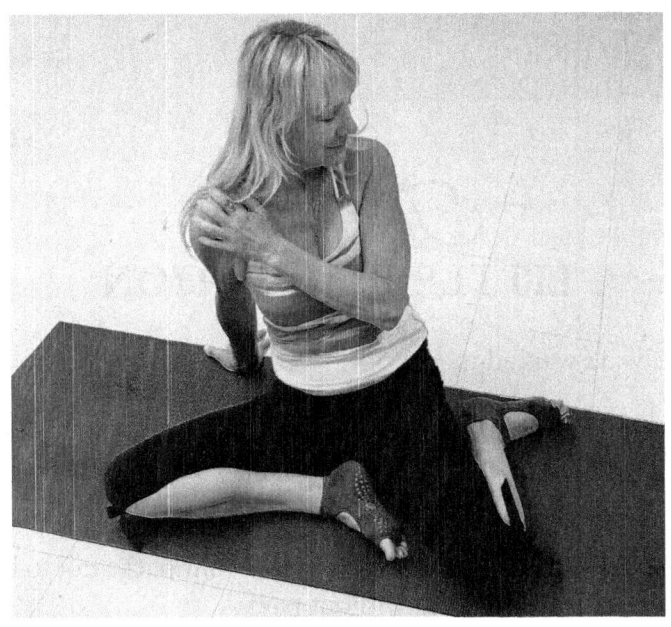

C. Rotate the head and shoulders in opposite directions (twisting motion) slowly 3 times

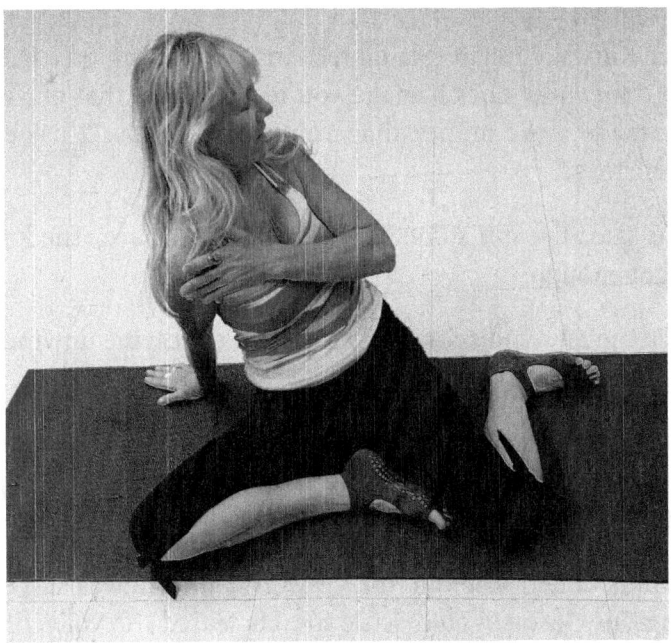

Perform the next two moves sitting the same way.

DAY TWENTY-SIX

The Dirty LITTLE TEMPTATION

We have always wanted more.

Whether it was a house, more kids, or just a single relationship that worked. We wanted a better job, more money, and to look better in the blue outfit.

Sometimes, it was very personal. We wanted our backs not to hurt or to be able to walk across a room without pain.

For those with power, to win another war or lift another trophy.

Always more.

The writer Kurt Vonnegut (Slaughterhouse Five) needled a friend once at a party, "Joe, how does it make you feel to know that our host only yesterday made more money than your novel Catch-22 has earned in its entire history?"

His friend said, "I've got something he can never have. The knowledge that I've got enough."

That's pretty great. And spoken from within the divine unwind.

We look at successful people or healthy people and think they must be happy. They must feel so good about themselves, what they've accomplished, what they have, the fact that they have no pain. Of course, it's not remotely true.

Tiger Woods called enough the "e-word", like it was an expletive, something only losers would settle for. He feared the void if he wasn't dominating the game. So, he played through injuries and against doctors' orders, doing serious damage to his body that follows him to this day.

Others who are pain-free know no joy, because they don't know what pain is.

Now, compare that to the stillness that comes from a sense of "enough". No relentless wanting. No insecurity of comparison. No need to do or have what you don't possess.

A place of love and stillness. What really matters.

Of course, no one will enjoy the magic sacredness of the divine unwind without a desire to get better and to become healthier. You must have a desire to improve and to grow and shed your pain along the way.

Yet, when it becomes insatiable, the desire for a pain-free life may disconnect you with other things in your life which are important.

Having enough comes from the inside. It comes from seeing yourself and your life differently, from knowing that more is not always the answer.

"When you realize there is nothing lacking," Lao Tzu says, "the whole world belongs to you."

If you can embrace this from within the divine unwind, you'll be richer than any billionaire. You may have less, but you'll have so much more.

Unwind to when you were young.

When I was a child, I had enough. I played in cardboard boxes and made necklaces out of flowers. I played with trucks in the dirt with my brother. Everything in the world was mine. I was rich.

MOVEMENT

SPANISH DANCER~ HEAD NOD

Staying to the right place both hands on the floor in front of your knee.

A. Tilt your head up and down 3 times slowly.

B. Tilt your head up with your eyes down 3 times

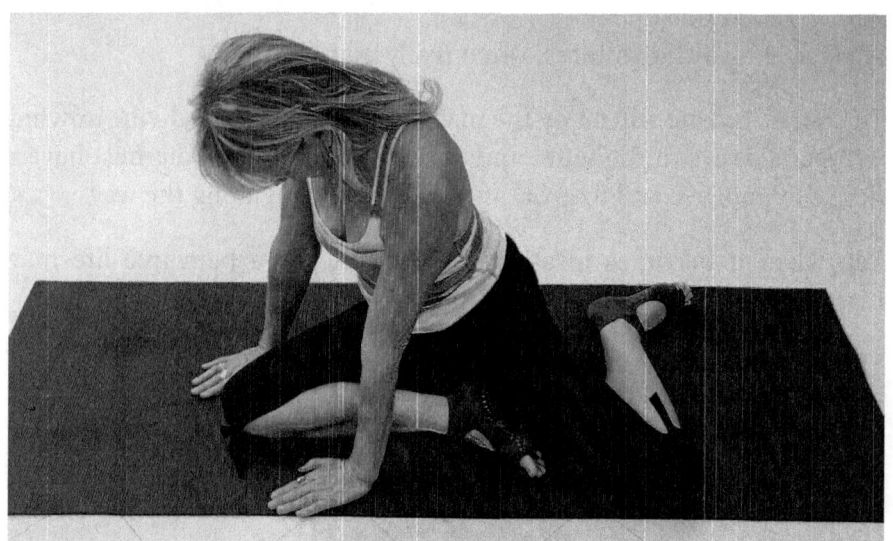

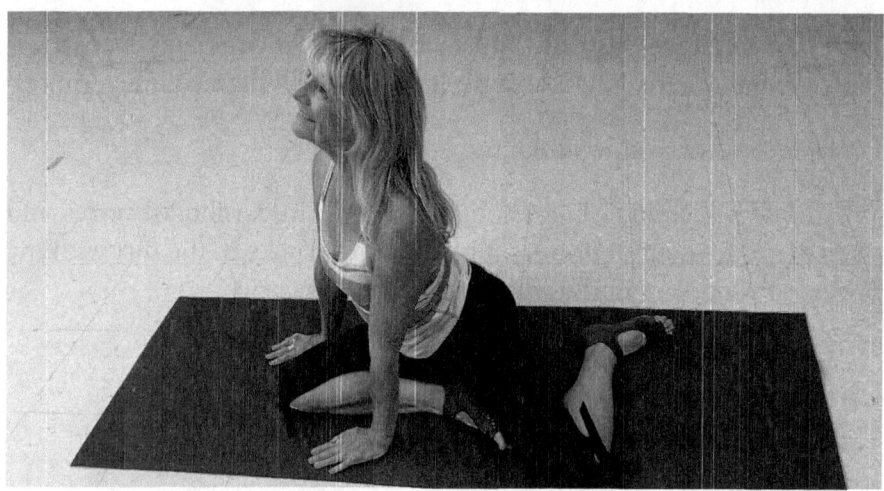

C. Place the left hand on the right shoulder, bring the elbow up with the head and eyes nodding downward and then bring the elbow down with the head and eyes nodding upward.

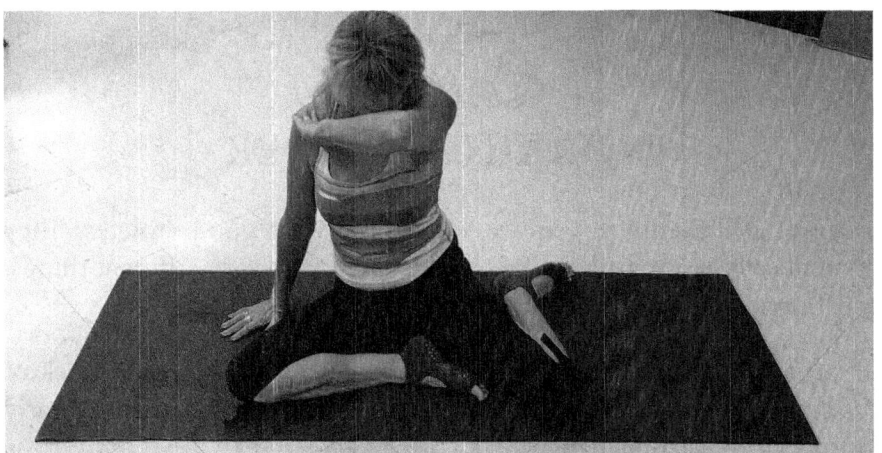

D. Right hand on the floor. Rotate the head to the left and keep it there, tilt the head upward while raising the shoulder up and bring them down together. Repeat 3 times.

Head nod with elbow lift.

A. Place the right hand on the left shoulder.

B. Tilt the head and eyes downward as the elbow goes up.

C. Switch slowly the right hand to the right shoulder, and, then, back to the left shoulder.

D. Keep the hand on the right shoulder, lift the elbow up and down, tilting the head up and down. Be creative with the eyes and head and elbow.

DAY TWENTY-SEVEN

Resting by WORKING HARDER

Some of my clients remember when they were good athletes. They remember that, for athletes, rest and recovery are very different things, a distinction that can help us with our divine unwind.

If you ask any serious runner how they recover from a hard week of running, their answer may surprise you: "I recover by going for an early morning run."

Yes, after exhausting themselves by running sixty miles in a week, runners recover by running more. This is a standard practice among top runners, and as crazy as it sounds, it works.

Too much time spent resting can actually make us more tired than before we started.

In the same way, we can recover our energy by strategically practicing active recovery, which looks a lot different from doing nothing.

Rest is passive. Too much time spent resting can actually make us more tired than before we started. No one's raring to go after a long TV binge. Hah. You can hardly get up.

Recovery is active. Unlike rest, recovery is an active and deliberate practice. Effective recovery means recovering the energy source that drives you, and that can only be done deliberately.

Abraham Lincoln said, "Give me six hours to chop down a tree, and I will spend the first four sharpening the axe."

To live out your divine unwind effectively, you should deliberately take time to renew and recover your sense of purpose, which is the foundation upon which day-to-day work is built.

Recovery is imperative for an effective unwind, because it is a form of perpetual preparation that allows us to focus on what matters to us. It can be done at the end of the day, but also at the beginning.

Journaling is one of the most effective way to manage your recovery. Journaling can have a positive effect on your emotional well-being. It's also a valuable tool for recovery.

Journaling is a re-cover of the day, a reflection on where you've been, and it helps you analyze whether your day-to-day actions are aligning with your motivations and intentions to unwind.

Writing out your thoughts will become, for many of you, a deliberate practice of honesty that will provide the narrative for your sacred journey.

If you only rest, the exterior may look attractive, but the interior won't be very nice, and it may even collapse. Rest and recovery are different, but both are essential to the divine unwind.

Listen to your body.

Unwind to when you were young.

I don't ever remember being tired ever when I was young. Like never.

MOVEMENT

SPANISH DANCER~HEAD TILT

Remain in the same position and take some weight off of the right hand by bringing it closer to you. Place your left hand over the top of your head, tilt your right ear towards your right shoulder and then tilt towards your left shoulder 3 times.slowly. Do not pull on your head. Grab your left ear lobe, gently tug it down tilting your head to the left 3 times.

Rotate all the way to the right, notice if you can see farther than when you started?

Repeat on the other side.

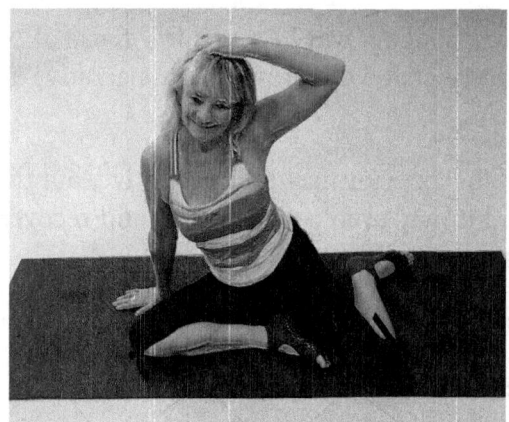

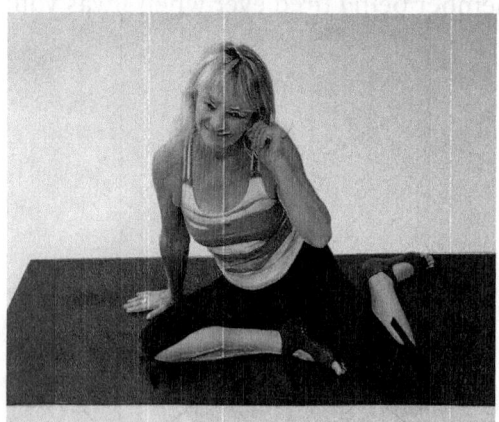

DAY TWENTY-EIGHT

Pandiculation

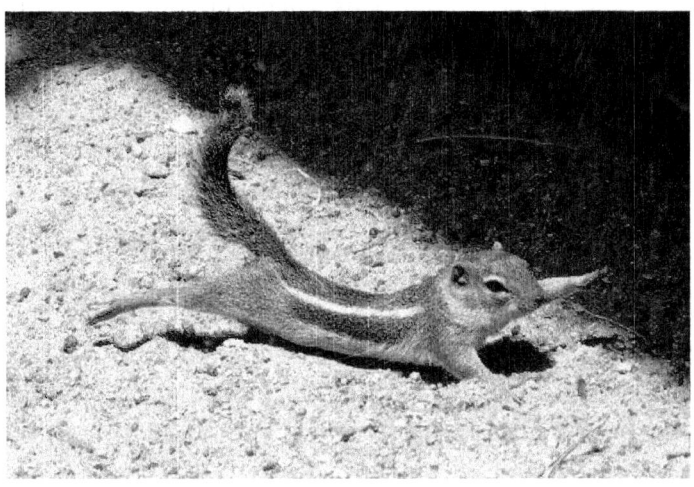

To PANDICULATE is to yawn and stretch at the same time.

Studies have shown that this actually exhilarated the muscles and stimulates alertness. Pandiculations are what animals do naturally in the wild. They pandiculate seven to eight times per day. They do not strive, stress, or worry as we do, and do not store trauma. The organic movements they perform daily prevent trauma and habitual contraction in their bodies.

Whereas children move all day long, reeducating the nervous system and brain, and keeping the muscles limber, flexible, resilient, and strong.

Somatic movements are not stretches. They are pandiculations, and perfectly safe to perform before exercise to correct postural alignment and for optimal performance.

STRESS is a huge factor in our lives, if we are to manage it, this is the best way I have found.

Let's plug that into your divine unwind. It's probably true that you are on stress overload. Of course, we want to mitigate that stress however possible. But as we unwind, how you feel about your stress may be more important than the stress, itself.

Is the pain related to the emotions? Absolutely. If I am depressed, it may depress my chest, shoulders sink in, and my jaw tightens, my abdominals get squished and all the insides. This will eventually cause pain.

Let's eliminate as much as possible the stress that is pain-related. See what can be done to solve the depression. Find what makes you sparkle again. When I go listen to music, I light up. It stimulates positive energy and, in turn, I feel better.

When I dance, I have no pain. It disappears.

My friend Charla is a dancer. She has had severe knee pain lately and is doing what she can somatically to relieve the tight muscles around her knee. She made a miraculous discovery: when she would dance, she had no pain, and the more she danced, the more the pain dissipated.

Remember that walking is the opposite of dancing.
When the foot lands in walking it is heel, ball, toe.
When you jog it is toe, ball, heel.
When you run it is heel, ball, toe.
When you dance, you dance on the ball of the foot, or in most dances toe, ball, heel.
The toe, ball, heel action is easier on the knee.
If you articulate the foot slowly, you can retrain the foot muscles as well.
Remember we have unlimited potential for learning in this area.
We can retrain the feet, hands, facial muscles to look younger, etc.

Use the many suggestions in this book and unwind to a thoughtful place of contemplation in considering relationships that need work.

I can feel you and love you. I want to grow young with you. When we meet, let's do a dance—not alone, but together.

Unwind to when you were young.

I remember, when I was young, I thought the best thing in the whole world was to be a grown-up and could not wait.

Had that wrong. Being young was the best.

MOVEMENT

ROLL UP

Sense; Standing, close your eyes and notice how you feel. Notice where your head is in space compared to your shoulders and feet. Notice any tention in the body. Notice where your weight is in your feet. front, back, inside, outside?

A. Roll down to touch your toes. Notice how far you are reaching down with your legs straight.

B. Roll up one vertebrae at a time and arch your back supporting your back with your hands. Notice how far you are looking back.

C. Roll down with your knees bent and up 3 times very slowly, one vertebrae at a time.

D. End reaching down with legs straight. Notice how far you are reaching

Sense; Roll up slowly keep the head tilted down and let the body come up to neutral, the head comes up last. Imagine a golden cord holding your head upright. Notice if your are more grounded into your heals. Notice where your head is in space. Sense and feel if the body is more comfortable or has less stress.

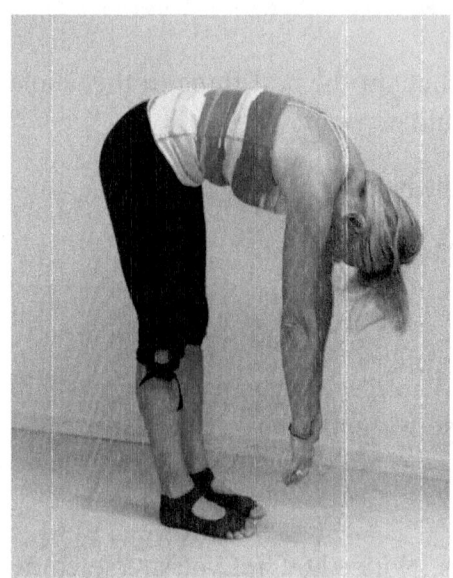
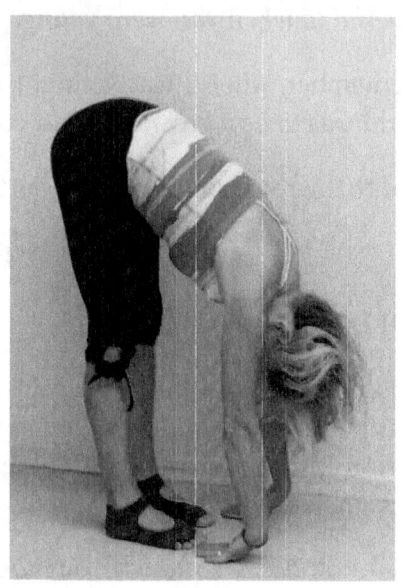
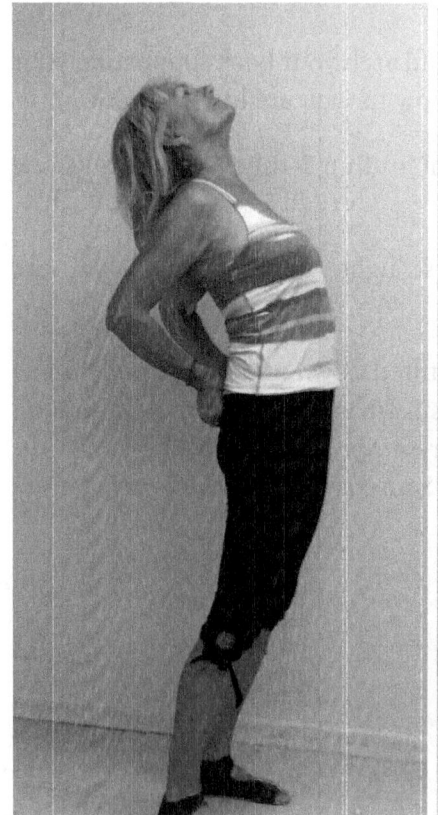
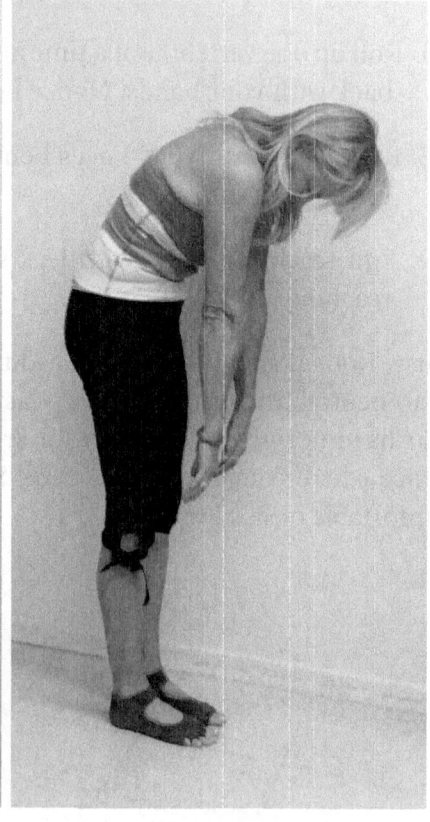

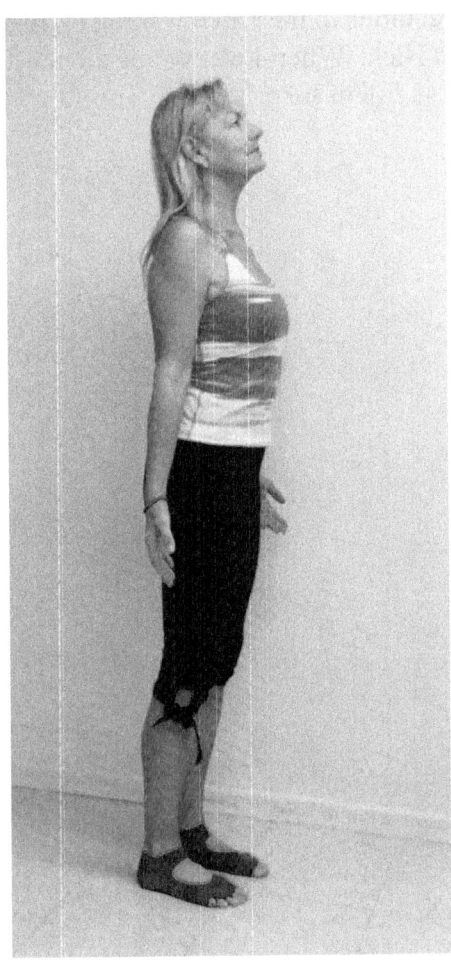

Hold your head up high, lift your belly button, feel the weight of your body into your heels, grounding you, keeping you rooted. Without this golden cord, your head may slump, and your feet may shuffle as you journey down your path today. Lift your perspective to a higher one with a heavenly view.

Unwind to when you were young.

I thought Christmas was a miracle. Lighting the candles at church at midnight, reading the story of christ being born and the angels and animals all gathered around.

It was all very miraculous to me. Then waking up to the presents under the tree from Saint Nick. When I was young all new things seemed like miracles. Life was so full of surprises.

DAY TWENTY-NINE

Miracles Are The
EVERYDAY STUFF OF GOD

When you're reading these words to this beautiful Fleetwood Mac song. Put your younger self in there.

> *I've been searching for a pot of gold.*
> *Like the kind you find at the end of the rainbow.*
> *I've been dreaming, thought it was in vain,*
> *ah but now you're here can't believe that your back again.*
> *And I know I can't lose, as long as you follow.*
> *I'm gonna win as long as you follow.*
> *I've been wandering gone away too far,*
> *But road was long to get back to where you are.*
> *And the sun went down, never seemed to rise,*
> *ah but now your here with the light shining in your eyes.*
>
> . *"As long as you follow"*
> **Fleetwood Mac**

We're all searching for that pot of gold. I found the miracle in this unwinding work. You can, too. Search for it like hidden treasure, and you will find it.

It's a miracle after all my accidents that I'm alive today to teach this to you. The somatic healing is a natural miracle. It was a miracle I wasn't harmed when I ran away from home at ten years old. It was a miracle I was protected when I hitchhiked in my teens and rode a motorcycle to and from work on Highway 17 from Santa Cruz to San Jose for a whole year in my twenties. It's also a miracle I lived through a head on collision at 50 miles an hour, serious head injury, and broken bones.

I am a miracle.

Wait for it.

Search for it.

The miracle is about to unfold.

Unwind to when you were young.

I remember sitting on a mound of seashells for hours looking for treasures.

MOVEMENT

STANDING DISHRAG

Stand with legs in a wide stance.
Bring arms out wide as well.
Rotate in opposite directions, rotating the head as well, slowly a few times.
Rotate the arms and head in opposite directions, looking past your shoulder.
Bring the arms up to one side and swoop down and up to the other side a few times.
Take the arms up and over the head like a rainbow to the other side and down, up over your head again, making a rainbow shape and down again a few times.

Enjoy the journey.

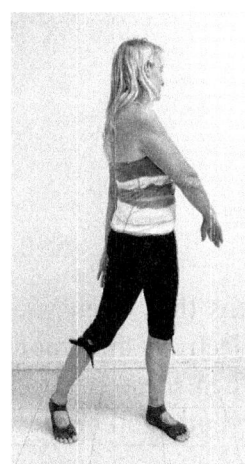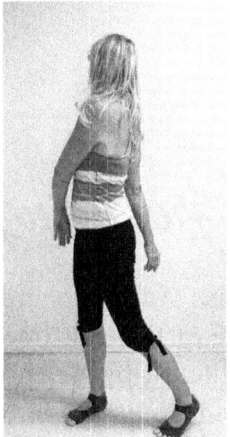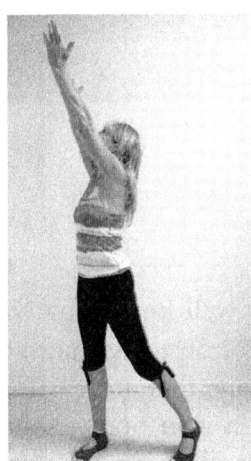

DAY THIRTY

Grounding

It was well known by Native American Indians that when you walk barefoot on the ground, the earth sends free electrons into your body. Electrons that are part of the earth, itself. When these electrons run through your body, it spreads to tissues in the body and creates some very good effects, relieving tension and stress.

Apparently, it has been rediscovered.

Check out *earthing.com*

The Indians wear moccasins made out of leather, a shoe that keeps you connected to the earth. There is something about being close to nature that really does relieve one's stress.

So what is grounding?

Grounding—also called earthing—is simply taking off your shoes and walking barefoot on the ground and feeling the earth and nature beneath your feet. In the days of Native America, the medicine man had this remedy at his beck and call.

There are some things to know about our earth. Rubber or plastic-soled shoes will not ground you to the earth. Leather shoes, however, do. You can walk on grass, soil, earth, sand, and also on concrete and ceramic tile. Another of the benefits is that walking on the earth barefoot (or with leather shoes) allows the body to get rid of the excess charge in your body. In this modern day, when every store has electronic equipment scanning you from head to foot as you enter and even walk around a store, not to mention all the wireless equipment in our homes and offices, this grounding is so needed.

Truly, God has given us everything we need for life, as the Bible says in 2 Peter 1:3.

So, the next time you're at the beach, stand on the wet sand, and if you're there long enough, you can feel this energy accumulating in your feet, ankles, and, then, your calves. It begins to move up the legs, reenergizing you from the ground up. I have experienced it myself, and it's an amazing feeling. I even found a small piece of earth in my courtyard to have lunch and put my feet on the wet, damp dirt while I'm eating. I could feel the energy rising up from within me.

Try it for yourself whenever you can take off your shoes and sense the earth beneath you. Wait for it…

You, too, will be amazed.

MOVEMENT

WALKING WARM UP

Stand in walking pattern stance, with feet hip width apart, and a comfortable stride length.

Rock back and forth with the weight on the front leg the back heal goes up like you are pushing off with your back foot. Weight on the back leg the toes go up in front mimicking the heal strike.

Swing the arms in counter balance. Keep your head up and looking at the horizon, not at the floor.

This Movement will help loosen up the muscles for walking.

Repeat about 10 to 20 times

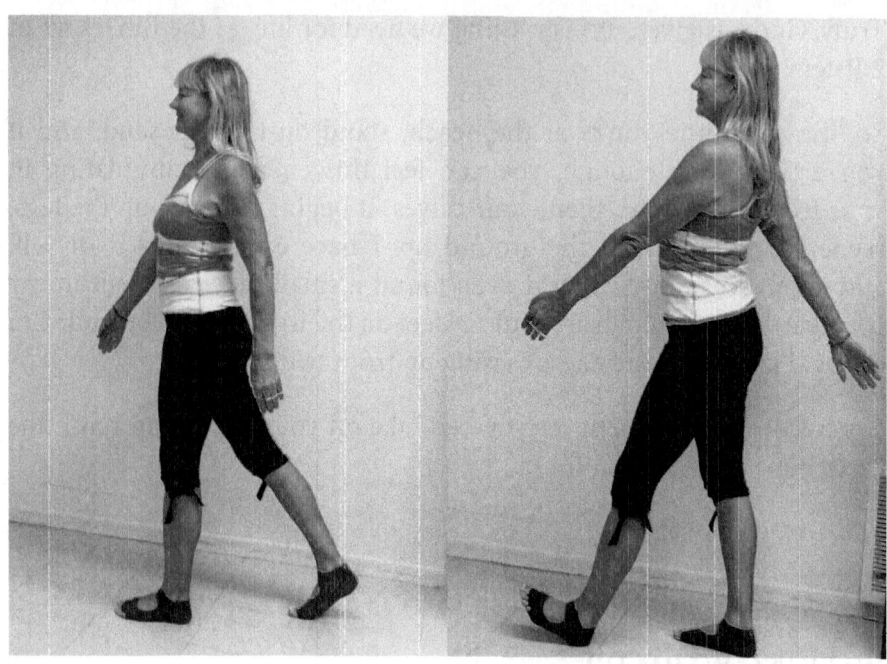

This warmup is great before walking. You are reminding the ankles and feet the bi pedal locomotion pattern we learned as a child. It improves balance and reestablishes a smoother walking pattern.

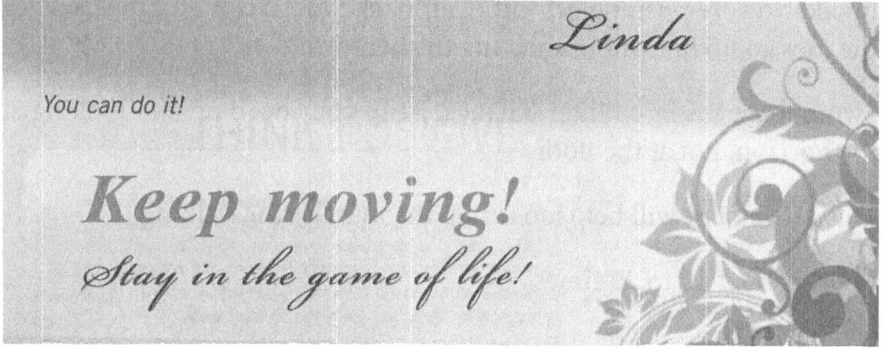

You can do it!

Linda

Keep moving!
Stay in the game of life!

I will always be dancing in the moonlight and under the stars, hopefully with you soon. Come out and sing and dance with me, or just play in the sand and the sun. We will grow young together and prove Thomas Hanna right that aging really is just a myth.

This song has a piece of my heart .

A Little Longer

*What can I do for you, what can I bring to you.
What kind of song would you like me to sing.
Cause I'll dance a dance for you
Pour out my love for you
What can I do for you, beautiful King.
Cause I can't thank you enough
With all of the words that I write,
I can't thank you enough, I pour out my life.
I can't thank you enough.
Then, I hear you say
You don't have to do a thing
Simply be with me and let those things go.
They can wait another minute,
Wait, this moment is too sweet,
Please stay here with me
And love on me a little longer,
Cause I'm in love with you.*

Bethel Music

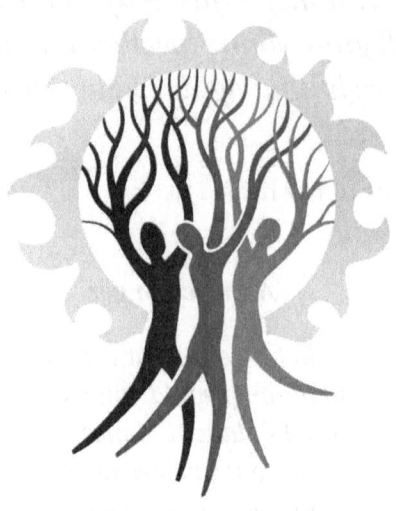

Website: *somaticlife.com*

E-mail: *somalinda@gmail.com*

More Movements to come in future books.

DVD of the Movement in this book filmed at the peaceful Lake San Marcos.

Subscribe to Linda Anna's You Tube Channel to somatize, dance, and earth with her.

Subscribe to her monthly newsletter to receive movement of the month and current videos.

Connect with her on **Facebook** and **Instagram**.

Follow me and like me.

Printed by BoD"in Norderstedt, Germany